THE SNOWS OF OLYMPUS

THE SNOWS OF OLYMPUS

A GARDEN ON MARS

ARTHUR C. CLARKE

VICTOR GOLLANCZ

LONDON

Dedicated
To the memory of 'Spark' Matsunaga
US Senator for Hawaii
and to
the first Martians – today's students of
the International Space University

First published in Great Britain 1994
by Victor Gollancz
A Division of the Cassell group
Villiers House, 41/47 Strand, London WC2N 5JE

A catalogue record for this book is
available from the British Library.

ISBN 0 575 05652 5

Designed by Stephen Bray
Typeset in Great Britain at The Spartan Press Ltd, Lymington, Hants
Printed and bound in Spain

Contents

MARS/EARTH VITAL STATISTICS

	Mars	Earth
Distance from Sun	228Mkm	150Mkm
Length of year	687 (Earth) days	364 days
Length of day	24h 40m	24h
Diameter	6787km	12,765km
Inclination	24°	23°
Gravity	371cm/sec^2	981cm/sec^2
Atmospheric pressure	7mb	1000mb
Atmospheric composition	CO_2 97 per cent	N_2 78 per cent
	N_2 3 per cent	O_2 21 per cent
Temperature	+10 to –120°C	+40 to –50°C
Number of moons	2	1

Prologue

A Message to Mars

The Explorers Club of New York has hosted many historic press conferences, but few could have been as unusual as the one which took place on 22 June 1993. On that day the Planetary Society's president, Carl Sagan, announced 'Visions of Mars', a project mounted in conjunction with the Time-Warner Interactive Group to send a gift 'from our era to the future generations of humans who will one day explore, and perhaps settle, Mars'.

To quote from the Society's Press Release:

Visions of Mars will be a collection of science-fiction stories, sounds and images on a compact disk that chronicle humanity's fascination with Mars and its imagined Martians from H. G. Wells to the present day. A copy of the disk will be placed inside each of the two small stations that *Mars 94** will land on the surface of the red planet in September, 1995 . . . Future recipients of the disks will find them in protected locations inside the small landers. A label on the exterior of each lander will announce in five languages the presence of the disk and how to play it . . . **Visions of Mars** will contain the equivalent of several thousand pages of fiction from writers around the world, from H. G. Wells to Isaac Asimov, Alexei Tolstoi to Kurt Vonnegut . . .

The disk will also include a portion of the Orson Welles radio broadcast of *War of the Worlds* . . . an audio recording made the night that the *Viking* 1 lander made the first successful landing on Mars, featuring reactions from Gene Roddenberry, Robert Heinlein, Ray Bradbury and others; and brief messages to the future inhabitants of Mars from key figures . . .

I felt extremely honoured by a request to make my own video contribution, though, considering the rate of obsolescence of audiovisual equipment on this planet, I could not help wondering if the New Martians will have the equipment to view it. Some time in the next century, however, I hope that these words will be heard on Mars:

My name is Arthur Clarke, and I am speaking to you from the island of Sri Lanka, once known as Ceylon, in the Indian Ocean, Planet Earth. It is early spring in the year 1993, but this message is intended for the future. I am addressing men and women – perhaps some of you already born – who will listen to these words when they are living on Mars.

As we approach the new millennium, there is great interest in the planet which may be the first real home for mankind beyond the mother world. During my lifetime, I have been lucky enough to see our knowledge of Mars advance from almost complete ignorance – worse than that, misleading fantasy – to a real understanding of its geography and climate. Certainly we are still very ignorant in many areas, and lack knowledge which you take for granted. But now we have accurate maps of your wonderful world, and can imagine how it might be modified – terraformed – to make it nearer to the heart's desire. Perhaps you are already engaged upon that centuries-long process.

There is a link between Mars and my present home, which I used in what will probably be my last novel, *The Hammer of*

*The first Russian *Mars* lander is due to be launched in October 1994, arriving in August 1995; a second, in 1996, will carry a 'Rover' as well as an instrument-carrying helium balloon. The projects are being carried out in close cooperation with NASA: however, the precarious economic situation in the former USSR – not to mention that in the present United States – make these schedules rather uncertain.

God [1993]. At the beginning of this century, an amateur astronomer named Percy Molesworth was living here in Ceylon. He spent much time observing Mars, and now there is a huge crater, 175km wide, named after him in your southern hemisphere. In my book I've imagined how a New Martian astronomer might one day look back at his ancestral world, to try and see the little island from which Molesworth – and I – often gazed up at your planet.

There was a time, soon after the first landing on the Moon in 1969, when we were optimistic enough to imagine that we might have reached Mars by the 1990s. In another of my stories ['Transit of Earth', 1971], I described a survivor of the first ill-fated expedition, watching the Earth in transit across the face of the Sun on May 11 – *1984*! Well, there was no one on Mars then to watch that event – but it will happen again on 10 November 2084. By that time I hope that many eyes will be looking back towards the Earth as it slowly crosses the solar disc, looking like a tiny, perfectly circular sunspot. And I've suggested that we should signal to you then with powerful lasers, so that you will see a star beaming a message to you from the very face of the Sun.

I too salute you across the gulfs of space – as I send my greetings and good wishes from the closing decade of the century in which mankind first became a spacefaring species, and set forth on a journey that can never end, so long as the Universe endures.

Introduction

This book is really an act of homage – a fond recollection of childhood dreams which I have seen achieved beyond all expectation. It is also a tribute to the men and women who shared those dreams: though most of them are now gone, I hope they will live again in these pages.

It is impossible for anyone born since the opening of the Space Age to understand what mystery and magic the very word 'Mars' once evoked. Yet both these qualities, I am happy to say, still remain in ample measure; though the canals have evaporated and Deja Thoris, Princess of Helium, has joined H. G. Wells' tentacled monstrosities in some alternate universe, the *real* Mars has proved to be almost as wonderful as the imaginary versions. And I have no doubt that the biggest surprises are yet to come.

I would like to have called this book *The Greening of Mars*, but Michael Allaby and James ('Gaia') Lovelock very unsportingly pre-empted that title almost a decade before I thought of it. A good alternative would have been *Green Mars*, but by another unlikely coincidence that is the name of an excellent story by Kim Stanley Robinson – published back-to-back with my own novella *A Meeting With Medusa* (1988) and now part of a massive trilogy. Clearly, there is a conspiracy afoot.

So I have stolen my subtitle from Pierre Boulle, best known for *The Bridge on the River Kwai* (1952; trans 1954). During the pre-*Apollo* year 1964, Boulle published a witty and entertaining novel, *Le jardin de Kanashima* (trans 1965), about the first Japanese astronaut on the Moon. This led to a confrontation between us when the French television channel TF1 telecast *Starglider: Portrait d'Arthur Clarke*. Details will be found in my 'sciencefictional autobiography' *Astounding Days* (1989); suffice it to say that the final score was Boulle 1, Clarke 1. So I had no hesitation in adapting Pierre's (translated) title, *A Garden on the Moon*.

Imagine my astonishment, several months later, to come across a photograph entitled 'Lowell gardening on Mars'! It appears in William Graves Hoyt's biography *Lowell and Mars*

(1976), and shows the present that the observatory staff gave the creator of the canal legend on his fiftieth birthday. They had pasted, on a globe of Mars, a photo of Lowell diligently modifying a piece of planet Earth with a small rake.

We will need considerably more massive equipment to 'garden' Mars. But, if they decide to do so, our descendants can create a New Earth – perhaps even a New Eden – on the next

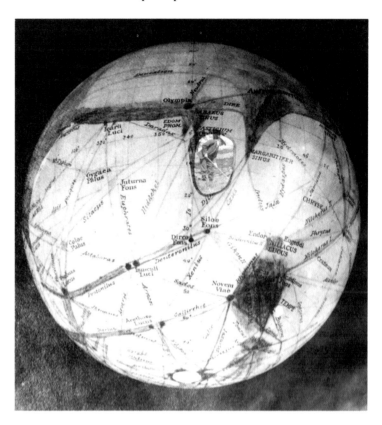

Percival Lowell 'gardening' on Mars! This Mars globe, with the photograph attached, was presented to Lowell by the observatory staff on his fiftieth birthday, 13 March 1905. (*Lowell Observatory Photograph*)

world outwards from the Sun. That is the main theme of this book.

It resulted from the fusion of three totally disparate elements, which unexpectedly combined in a way that now seems inevitable. And it all happened in a single day; the concept exploded in my head one morning, and by nightfall the synopsis was complete. The first two components were Pasadena's Jet Propulsion Laboratory and the Big Island of Hawaii – places I have been fortunate enough to visit in what our century may be the last to call 'real' life. The third ingredient is something which,

until recently, existed only in science fiction. In my younger days, I sometimes fantasized that I would visit the Moon – but I never imagined that I would explore Mars! Now, thanks to the astonishing developments in personal computers and virtual-reality software, I am able to do just that.

And so can you. Fasten your seatbelts.

ARTHUR C. CLARKE
Chancellor, International Space University
Colombo, Sri Lanka, September 1993

OPPOSITE: **A glaciated vista of Mars, with the glaciers seeming out of place among the volcanic craters. Ironically, this scene could be either from Mars' distant past – perhaps several million years ago – or from its not-quite-so-distant future, in perhaps a few hundred thousand years' time, when a new ice age has created glaciers from the water released millennia before by terraforming.** (*Painting by Michael Carroll, reproduced by permission*)

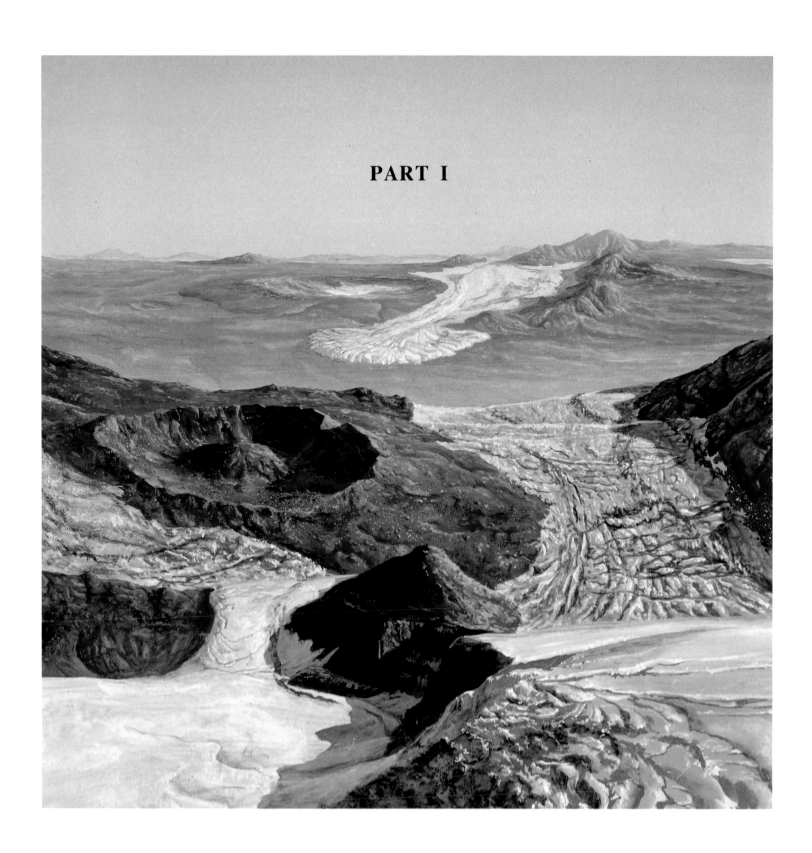

PART I

1

Prelude to Mars

Viewed under suitable conditions, few sights can compare for instant beauty and growing grandeur with Mars as presented by the telescope. Framed in the blue of space, there floats before the observer's gaze a seeming miniature of his own Earth, yet changed by translation to the sky. Within its charmed circle of light he marks apparent continents and seas, now ramifying into one another, now stretching in unique expanse over wide tracts of the disc, and capped at their poles by dazzling ovals of white . . .

. . . And very vivid are the tints, so salient and so unlike that their naming in words conveys scant idea of their concord to the eye. Rose ochre dominates the lighter regions, while a robin's-egg blue colours the darker; and both are set off and emphasized by the icy whiteness of the caps . . . In some parts of the light expanses the ochre prevails alone; in others the rose deepens to a brick-red, suffusing the surface with the glow of a warm, late afternoon . . .

So rhapsodized the US astronomer Percival Lowell in his *Mars as the Abode of Life* (1908), and this lyrical passage can serve as both inspiration and warning. At the very least it suggests that there was something peculiar about Lowell's eyesight: 'the *blue* of space', indeed!

Anyone who has never observed Mars through a telescope cannot imagine what a frustrating target the planet usually is. I flatly refuse to let my friends look at it (even through my 14in [36cm] Celestron) because disappointment is inevitable. Admittedly my locale in the middle of a large city is not the best observing site, but the last time I looked at Mars, though it was almost overhead, all I could see was a fuzzy pink disc showing no markings whatsoever. Not even the polar cap was visible.

At its very closest, Mars is only one-fiftieth the apparent diameter of the Moon. To the naked eye, the Moon shows a fair amount of detail, and a magnification of fifty is a very modest figure. So it might be thought that, even with a small instrument, one could see a good deal on an apparently Moon-sized Mars. Unfortunately, sheer magnifying power cannot help very

much. Unlike the Moon, the disc of Mars shows very little contrasting detail; *pace* Lowell, it is a mottled patchwork of subtle shades, merging imperceptibly into one another. The only really outstanding features are the polar caps, waxing and waning with seasons twice as long as Earth's.

To make matters even worse, when Mars is at its closest we lie directly between it and the Sun; as every amateur photographer knows, such lighting conditions give a 'flat' and often misleading image. While the Moon goes through its phases we can watch the long shadows sweep across plain and crater, and get a vivid – almost 3-D – impression of its topography, but if you look at the *full* Moon through any telescope (an ordinary pair of binoculars will suffice) it appears completely flat: you would never guess the existence of its magnificent mountain ranges. So it is with the full Mars: from our position closer to the Sun we can get a side view only when the planet is too far away for good observation. And although large telescopes can employ powers of several thousand – making Mars appear as big as a beachball at arm's-length – images magnified that much

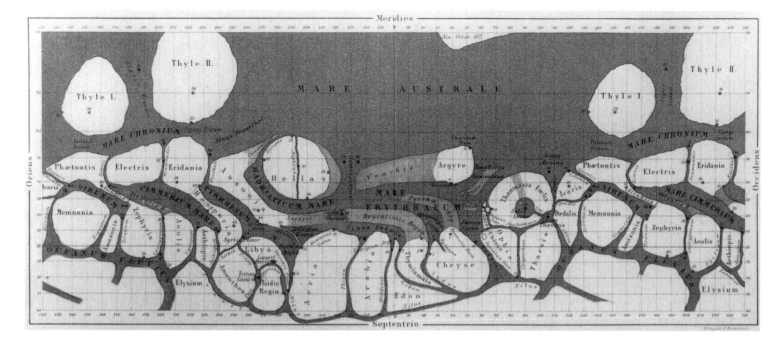

The map of Mars produced in 1877 by the Italian astronomer Giovanni Schiaparelli. Note that the 'channels' ('canali'), as Schiaparelli called them, do not look at all artificial – and, indeed, he himself never suggested that they were. (*Lowell Observatory Photograph*)

are so fuzzy as to be almost useless.* The Earth's atmosphere interposes a continually shifting veil between our eyes and the Universe around us. Even on the most crystal-clear night, astronomers are like fish trying to look at the strange world of dry land through the trembling interface of air and water.

This state of affairs gravely limited Mars studies until the opening of the Space Age, and was responsible for one of the strangest episodes in the entire history of astronomy – the Great Canal Delusion. It all began in 1877, with the mistranslation of one word, and lasted for almost a century.

Because the orbit of Mars is somewhat eccentric, its distance during its closest approach to Earth ('opposition') varies widely, ranging between fifty and one hundred million kilometres. An unusually favourable opposition occurred in 1877, so every astronomer interested in the planet took advantage of the exceptional close-up. One such was the US astronomer Asaph Hall, using a 26in (66cm) refractor at the US Naval Observatory in Washington. In August 1877 he discovered that Mars has two tiny moons, quickly named Phobos (Fear) and

Deimos (Panic) after the attendants of the Roman God of War.

Much more sensational, however, was the news from Milan, where the distinguished Italian astronomer Giovanni Schiaparelli reported that the planet appeared to be criss-crossed with a network of narrow lines. His 1877 map showed them as well defined bands or streaks, most running north–south. However, they were not particularly straight and certainly gave no impression of artificiality. Schiaparelli labelled them with the noncommittal name 'channels' (*canali*), but this was promptly translated into English as 'canals' – a word with altogether different resonances. Canals implied builders, and so the 'Martians' were born.

Their midwife – or at least their nurse – was the brilliant scion of a famous New England family. Thanks to the energy and literary skills of Percival Lowell, probably most of the world's reading public became acquainted with his ideas on Mars, though usually at second hand through sensational newspaper reports. When Schiaparelli reported his 'channels' in 1877,

*Recent developments in 'adaptive optics' and electronic imaging are overcoming these problems. Remarkable images of Mars have now been obtained with Earth-based telescopes; the Hubble Space Telescope, despite its initial problems, can do even better from its vantage point above the atmosphere.

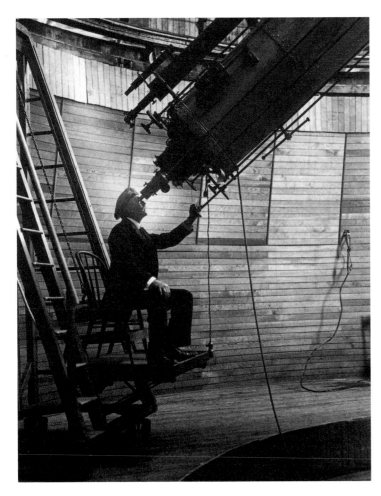

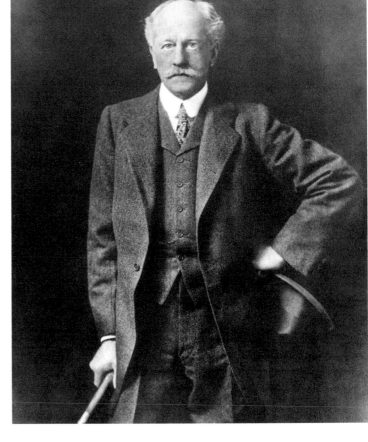

Lowell with the Flagstaff Observatory's 24in (610mm) refractor. Although this photograph was taken in daytime, he is actually using the telescope – to observe the planet Venus, which is often easily visible to the naked eye even in broad daylight. (*Lowell Observatory Photograph*)

Percival Lowell's own favourite picture of himself. The photograph must have been taken at about the beginning of this century. (*Lowell Observatory Photograph*)

Lowell was only twenty-two. He spent the next six years in the family business – running a cotton mill, managing trust funds and building up such a substantial fortune that before he was thirty he was able to do anything he wished. For the succeeding decade he travelled around the world, and became so fascinated by the Far East that he rented a house in Tokyo. After only three weeks in the country he wrote home: 'I am beginning to talk Japanese like a native (of America).' He was in fact a remarkable linguist – he had been fluent in French at ten and in Latin at eleven – and the head of the US Legation in Tokyo wrote that 'he has learned Japanese faster than I ever saw any man learn a language'. Lowell made such an impression on his compatriots that he was asked to lead the first US Mission to Korea, which he did with great success. If he had not turned to astronomy he could well have become a diplomat; indeed, he published more books about Japan and Korea than he ever did about Mars.

His oriental excursions ended when he was in his late thirties, and thereafter Mars dominated his life. In October 1894 the planet would make another of its closer approaches to the Earth

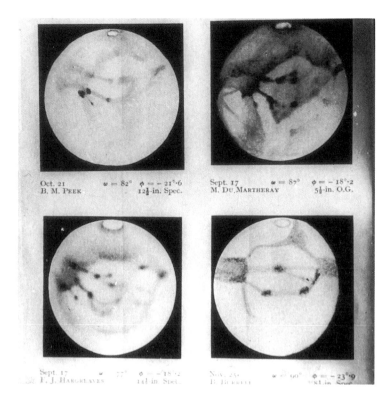

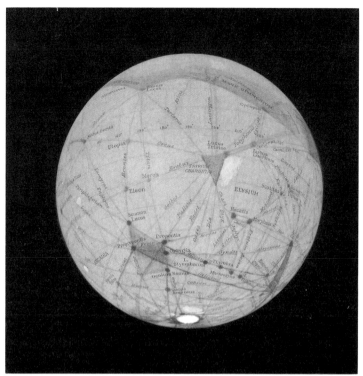

Accustomed as we are to high-resolution photographs of the Martian surface provided for us by space-probes, it is easy to forget that astronomers of the past, even using the best available telescopes, had to make do with maddeningly elusive images. These drawings, purportedly substantiating Lowell's hypothesis of an intelligent civilization peopling the red planet, are typical of the best views of Mars that astronomers had before the beginning of the Space Age. (*Lowell Observatory Photograph*)

This Lowellian globe of Mars was produced in 1903, the same year that saw the start of the Air Age. A globe of Earth showing the routes of today's major airlines would look equally artificial. (*Lowell Observatory Photograph*)

– and, as Schiaparelli and Hall had done seventeen years earlier, Lowell was determined to make the most of the opportunity. He decided to install the best telescope he could obtain (an excellent 24in [61cm] refractor) under the clearest possible skies. Lowell was one of the first astronomers to emphasize the vital importance of locating observatories at sites with the most perfect seeing, usually on high mountaintops. He chose Flagstaff, Arizona, at an altitude of over two kilometres, starting a trend that has continued to this day. But even the best terrestrial site still has half the atmosphere above it, and good seeing can never be guaranteed.

Imagine that you are looking at a tennis ball suspended several metres away, and that you are trying to make an accurate drawing of the faint smudges that someone has daubed

on it. That is essentially what Lowell and his assistants were trying to do during their observations of Mars. No wonder that, straining their eyes to record details at the very limits of vision – and beyond – they 'saw' features that existed only in their imaginations.

Lowell went to his grave in 1916 convinced that Mars was covered with a network of narrow lines, most of them following great circles, and many intersecting in dark spots which he christened 'oases' – because that is precisely what he thought they were. The charts he drew after two decades of observation bear an uncanny resemblance to something that did not exist until long after his death: a map of the Earth's airlines. No natural process could have produced patterns of such geometrical regularity. Whatever they were, they could only be artificial.

To quote Lowell's own words from *Mars* (1896):

We have been led to regard it probable that upon the surface of Mars we see the effects of local intelligence . . . There is an apparent dearth of water upon the planet's surface, and therefore, if beings of sufficient intelligence inhabited it, they would have to resort to irrigation to support life . . . there turns out to be a network of markings covering the disc precisely counterparting what a system of irrigation would look like; and lastly, there is a set of spots placed where we should expect to find the lands thus artificially fertilized, and behaving as such constructed oases should. All this, of course, may be a set of coincidences; but the probability points the other way . . . The evidence of handicraft, if such it be, points to a highly intelligent and scientific mind behind it. Irrigation, unscientifically conducted, would not give us such truly wonderful mathematical fitness in the several parts as we there behold. A mind of no mean order would seem to have presided over the system we see – a mind certainly of considerably more comprehensiveness than that which presides over the various departments of our own public works. Party politics, at all events, have had no part in them; for the system is planet-wide. Quite possibly, such Martian folk are possessed of inventions of which we have not dreamed, and with them electrophones and kinetoscopes are things of a bygone past, preserved with veneration in museums as relics of the clumsy contrivances of the simple childhood of the race. Certainly what we see hints at the existence of beings who are in advance of, not behind us, in the journey of life.

What a pyramid of speculation, on a basis which was not merely flimsy but completely nonexistent! The key phrases in Lowell's conclusion are 'we see the effects . . .', 'we there behold . . .', 'what we see . . .'. But only Lowell and his disciples were able to 'see' or 'behold' the planet-wide artefacts of the Martian engineers.

Even in Lowell's lifetime his observations came under attack by eminent astronomers with equally fine instruments in equally good locations. They reported that, when the atmosphere became stable for a few precious moments, they could see the disc of Mars crowded with so much detail that it was impossible for eye and brain to grasp it all. But in those rare instants of 'perfect' seeing there was no sign of the canals!

A partial explanation of this curious phenomenon was given in 1903 by the distinguished UK astronomer Walter Maunder.* His counter to the Lowellian fantasy was as simple as it was effective. He took a group of English schoolboys and asked them to copy a picture of Mars – from which all lines resembling canals had been carefully removed. Nevertheless, many of the resulting drawings showed linear markings, and Maunder concluded that the canals were due to 'the integration by the eye of minute details too small to be separately and distinctly defined . . . It seems a thousand pities that all those magnificent theories of human habitation, canal construction . . . and the like are based upon lines which our experiments compel us to declare nonexistent.'

There can now be no doubt that Maunder's explanation was correct, though Lowell predictably ridiculed what he called the 'Small Boy Theory'. But on one point the UK astronomer was grossly unfair to his US colleague. Time and again Lowell had made the point that any hypothetical Martians would not be remotely 'human', because they would have evolved under very different conditions of gravity, atmosphere and climate. He ended his book *Mars* with words which are perhaps even more valid now than when they were written a century ago:

If astronomy teaches anything, it teaches that man is but a detail in the evolution of the Universe, and that resemblant though diverse details are inevitably to be expected in the host of orbs around him. He learns that, though he will probably never find his double anywhere, he is destined to discover any number of cousins scattered through space.

While hosting the television series *The Mysterious World of Arthur C. Clarke* I took the opportunity of repeating Maunder's experiment, using the pupils of a leading girl's college in Trincomalee, the great port on the east coast of Sri Lanka. My little experiment was conducted at short notice, and was not done very scientifically. I drew a circle on a sheet of cardboard and covered it with a random assortment of blobs and smudges, being careful to avoid any obvious alignments. But, sure enough, some of the girls did produce very convincing canals. Maunder would have been proud of them.

*Maunder has achieved posthumous fame for his discovery of the 'Maunder minimum' in sunspot activity. He also, in 1882, observed one of the finest UFOs ever reported – a 'great circular disc of greenish light . . . that moved across the sky as smoothly and steadily as the Sun, Moon, stars and planets move, but nearly a thousand times as quickly.' It was, he later reminisced, the most remarkable sight he had ever witnessed in his entire career; but, being a good scientist, he was immediately able to establish its identity as part of a great auroral display.

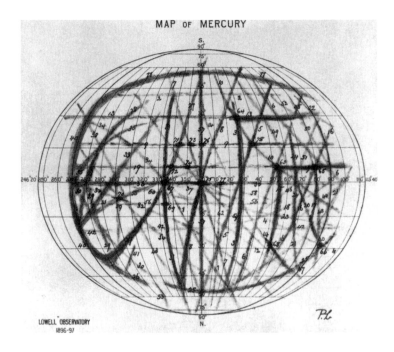

MAP OF MERCURY

LOWELL OBSERVATORY
1896-97

A map purporting to show the surface features of the planet Mercury, drawn up by Lowell in 1897. The linear markings show a distinct family resemblance to the Martian 'canals' – and are just as fictitious. In fact, as we now know, the surface of Mercury is a mass of overlapping craters with no distinctive overall features – very similar to the terrain in the most battered regions of the Moon. Since it is far, far harder to observe Mercury's surface from Earth than even that of Mars, even at the time this map must have seemed an imaginative exercise. (*Lowell Observatory Photograph*)

That there was something seriously wrong with Lowell's eyes was demonstrated beyond doubt by his later 'observations' of Mercury and Venus. His drawings of these are almost laughable, especially in view of what we now know about the two planets. The surface of Mercury closely resembles that of the Moon – flat, lava-covered plains and innumerable impact craters. Nevertheless Lowell drew a gridwork of intersecting lines, fuzzier than his gossamer-like Martian canals, but otherwise very similar. The fact that he had produced such drawings as early as 1897 makes it surprising that his later work on Mars was ever taken seriously. His 'chart' of Venus, made about the same time, is equally absurd. It too shows a pattern of linear features, rather like the spokes of a wheel, radiating from a central hub. Though Lowell was convinced that he was recording surface details, a series of space missions has now confirmed

what was long suspected – that Venus is covered with an atmosphere so thick (one hundred times denser than Earth's) that the surface can never be seen from space. The only genuine features that terrestrial astronomers have ever observed are temporary cloud formations; not until the advent of radar surveys was the truly bizarre surface of Venus – hot as the interior of a furnace – revealed. One day, perhaps, the human race may attempt the taming of what was once hopefully called Earth's sister world, but for the moment Mars is, by comparison, *already* a Garden of Eden.

Lowell's fantasy dominated – or at least influenced – the public image of Mars for almost half a century, and was the direct inspiration of countless works of fiction. The most famous was H. G. Wells' classic novel *The War of the Worlds* (1898), which became even more famous on Hallowe'en 1938 when Howard Koch and Orson Welles adapted it for radio. The resulting 'Panic Broadcast' was one of the first demonstrations of the new medium's power, and H. G. Wells was reported to be quite upset by the whole affair. However, all was forgiven by the time of his last visit to the United States, during which he met Welles in a San Antonio radio station on 28 October 1940:

Wells: Well, I've had a series of most delightful experiences since I came to America, but the best thing that has happened so far is meeting my little namesake here, Orson. I find him most delightful – he carries my name with an extra 'e' which I hope he'll drop soon . . . Are you *sure* there was such a panic in America, or was it your Hallowe'en fun?
Welles: I think that's the nicest thing that the man from England could possibly say about the man from Mars.

Despite being inevitably dated, Wells' *The War of the Worlds* retains much of its power: anyone who doubts that should listen to Richard Burton read its marvellous opening sentences in Jeff Wayne's musical version:

No one would have believed in the last years of the Nineteenth Century that this world was being watched keenly and closely by intelligences greater than man's yet as mortal as his own; that as men busied themselves about their various concerns they were scrutinized and studied, perhaps almost as narrowly as a man with a microscope might scrutinize the transient creatures that swarm and multiply in a drop of water . . . Yet across the gulf of space, minds that are to our minds as the beasts that perish, intellects vast and cool and unsympathetic, regarded this Earth with envious eyes, and slowly and surely drew their plans against us . . .

I wonder if even Wells could ever have dreamed that, in the last years of the twentieth century, men would be drawing up plans not *against* Mars, but *for* it . . .

Perhaps even more widely read than *The War of the Worlds* were the eleven novels, beginning with *A Princess of Mars* (1912–17), that Edgar Rice Burroughs set on a planet which clearly owed much to Lowell's speculations. Yet Burroughs added one brilliant touch which, as far as I know, was original: the 'atmosphere machine' which alone made life possible on his exotic but worn-out Barsoom. This was indeed a remarkable anticipation of terraforming.

I cannot leave the imaginary Mars without mentioning three other authors who have set their mark, and in one case his name, upon it. The first was the US writer Stanley G. Weinbaum, who burst upon the science-fiction scene like a nova with 'A Martian Odyssey' (*Wonder Stories*, 1934); alas, again like a nova, he was short-lived, dying of cancer little over a year after this first appearance. His memorial is an 82km crater in Mars' southern hemisphere.

C. S. Lewis used a somewhat Lowellian Mars as background for his theological speculations in *Out of the Silent Planet* (1938) before moving on to Venus in *Perelandra* (1943). Both novels are beautifully written, but many would-be astronauts were annoyed when Lewis attacked their visions of – as he called it – 'interplanetary imperialism'.

The last writer of distinction to be identified with an already habitable Mars is of course Ray Bradbury, whose 'Martian Chronicles' started appearing in 1946. Bradbury is, happily, still with us, but one day he will surely be posthumously honoured alongside Wells, Burroughs and Weinbaum with a crater on the planet which inspired their dreams.

The first glimpses of the real Mars began to appear in the 1965–76 period, when the *Mariner* space-probes flew past and the *Vikings* went into orbit and dropped landers. As the superbly detailed images flowed back from these probes to Earth, the ghosts of Lowell's canals – and their builders – were finally laid.

Or were they? In 1971 the US astronomer Dr Peter Boyce had a curious experience when observing Mars through one of the world's best telescopes, on a Chilean mountain under the finest conditions he had ever known. As he scanned Syrtis Major – one of the dark triangular markings usually to be seen on the planet's surface – he suddenly saw a classic Lowellian canal stretching from its pointed tip. As he watched in amazement, other markings appeared, including more lines and even 'oases'. He was absolutely certain about what he saw, although at the same time well aware of the *Mariner* photographs showing the absence of Martian canals. I believe his experience accounts for what happened to many of Lowell's contemporaries; it demonstrates the amazing ability of the eye–brain system to recreate images from memory.

Although I have never seen the canals of Mars, I am sure I could – if I tried hard enough.

The modern era is not, however, without its own popular fallacies concerning life on Mars.

On 25 September 1992 a Titan rocket lifted off from the Kennedy Space Center, Cape Canaveral, on the United States' first mission to Mars in two decades. *Mars Observer* was the most sophisticated spacecraft ever sent to the planet; it was due to go into a two-hour polar orbit, at a height of 380km, and then begin a survey of the planet lasting for two Earth years (1994–5) – or one complete Martian year of 687 Earth days. Although *Mars Observer* carried many scientific instruments for remote probing of the planet's atmosphere and mineral composition, most eagerly awaited were the images to be sent back by its onboard camera. Some of these would have had a resolution of only three metres, far surpassing anything sent back by *Mariner* or *Viking*. Alas, as the world knows, *Mars Observer* was lost in space, with devastating results not only to NASA (National Aeronautics and Space Administration) and JPL (the Jet Propulsion Laboratory at Houston) but to the many scientists who had devoted substantial fractions of their lives to its construction, and who had planned to spend even more years analysing the information it would have sent back to Earth.

To add insult to injury, some crackpot groups have suggested that NASA deliberately sabotaged *Mars Observer* to prevent it exposing a cover-up of some kind! I do not know the logic, if it can be called that, behind this theory: presumably NASA already knows that there *are* Martians, but for some strange reason has been concealing the fact. It is hard to think of any hypothesis that could be further from the truth: the slightest hint that there was life on Mars would have solved NASA's budget problems years ago.

Many of us had hoped that *Mars Observer* would settle once and for all the dispute over the notorious Mars Face. In some ways this affair is reminiscent of the Great Canal Controversy. However, there is one major difference: no one disputes that the Mars Face really exists, for it is present on two *Viking* images made thirty-five days apart. It is certainly an intriguing – even surprising – object, but can it be anything other than a natural formation, carved over the aeons by the random play of Martian dust-storms?

At least two books have been published suggesting that the Mars Face is not only artificial but is associated with a group of pyramids and other curious shapes to form what, for want of a better word, might be called a city. *Unusual Mars Surface Features* (1988) by V. DiPietro, G. Molenaar and J. Brandenburg contains numerous computer-massaged versions of the *Viking* images, one of which even appears to show *teeth* in the mouth of the slightly simian Face!

Richard C. Hoagland's *The Monuments of Mars: A City on the Edge of Forever* (1987) is a much more elaborate development of the theme, ranging widely over most of human culture, art and mythology in its speculations about the Face and its associated 'structures'. No brief summary can do it justice, but I cannot resist one quotation: 'And now here I was, gazing down on the ruins of a lost civilization on the Red Planet, thinking: "Of all the people who are *not* going to believe me, the first is Arthur Clarke."' My slightly-too-imaginative friend Dick Hoagland* is quite right; but I do not completely *dis*believe him, either. Had I been in charge of the *Mars Observer* program, the Cydonia region would have been one of my first priorities for a high-resolution scan. However, my coefficient of scepticism about an artificial origin for the Mars Face and the Martian Pyramids, originally about 99 per cent, has increased to 99.9 per cent as a result of two discoveries.

The first was that there is a 'Face' on Earth, too – and not just any old Face. Some years ago a Canadian air survey photographed a formation which was, quite unmistakably, a profile of George Bernard Shaw – and which was promptly named after him. It has been well asked: 'What strange powers did the Ancients possess, which enabled them to erect this monument to a famous playwright – thousands of years before he was born?'

*I owe him a considerable debt of gratitude. He was the first to suggest that life might exist in the ice-covered oceans of Jupiter's satellite Europa. See *2010: Odyssey Two* (1982).

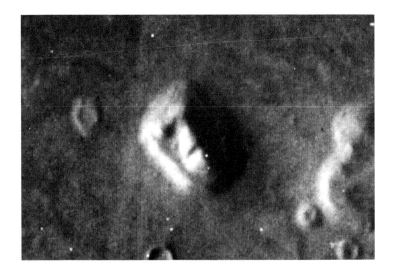

The famous Mars Face, first observed in *Viking* orbiter pictures in 1976 (this image is from *Viking* orbiter 1, frame 35A72). Perhaps it will be one of the great Martian tourist attractions of the twenty-first century, with some of the more credulous visitors from Earth *still* refusing to believe that it could be a natural formation! (*Photograph courtesy NASA/JPL*)

My curiosity about pyramids on Mars was terminally deflated one evening when I screened the restored version of David Lean's masterpiece *Lawrence of Arabia* (1962). Imagine my astonishment when I noticed that Peter O'Toole was racing his camel past an almost perfect *yet obviously natural* pyramid – and one considerably larger, as far as I could judge, than the manmade imitations at Giza!

So it appears that the combination of wind, sand and the other forces of erosion can produce all sorts of unexpected – indeed, at first sight impossible – results over the course of time. If this is true on Earth, it will certainly be true on Mars: in fact, when I examined the *Viking* images of the Cydonia region I kept discovering all sorts of vaguely humanoid faces popping out of the alien landscape. The Lowell Effect was hard at work again: I was finding what I was looking for.

In any event – a *human* face on Mars! How would that fit into the evolutionary sequence?

Easily, of course. We all know that the Atlanteans had spaceships. Or was it the Lemurians?

2

The Curtain Rises

On 12 November 1971 four incurable Mars-addicts met at Pasadena's famous Jet Propulsion Laboratory: Carl Sagan, Ray Bradbury, Bruce Murray (later to become JPL's Director) and myself. Under the chairmanship of the *New York Times'* distinguished science editor Walter Sullivan, we conducted a free-ranging discussion before a large and enthusiastic audience. The timing was impeccable. Next day, *Mariner* 9 was due to go into orbit round Mars and conduct the first detailed reconnaissance of the planet.

Three US spacecraft – *Mariners* 4, 6 and 7 (*Mariner* 5 went to Venus) – had been to Mars during the preceding six years with, from a romantic's point of view, frankly disappointing results. They had radioed back images of a flat landscape peppered with impact craters, almost indistinguishable from the lunar surface. Between them the three *Mariners* had returned about 200 images, covering a mere ten per cent of the planet. Ironically – as if Mars were keeping its secrets to the end – that ten per cent chanced to be the most unexciting part of a world with a total *land* surface almost the same as Earth's. Of course, we did not know this happenstance on the eve of the *Mariner* 9 encounter, and, though there were occasional flashes of optimism, few of us had very high hopes for the mission, even if everything worked perfectly. We expected to see more of the same dreary, flat terrain, pockmarked with innumerable craters.

Nevertheless, the discussion (later published as *Mars and the Mind of Man* [1973]) was great fun. Sagan gave a summary of what little was known and what much was speculated about the planet. In particular, he contrasted the wild fantasies of Percival Lowell with the amazingly accurate conclusions drawn by Alfred Russel Wallace.* In his book-length review of Lowell's theories, *Is Mars Habitable?* (1908), Wallace gave them a resounding 'no!', for reasons which we now know to be perfectly valid.

*Co-discoverer of the principle of evolution by natural selection and the man who jump-started the dilatory Darwin into publishing *The Origin of Species* (1859).

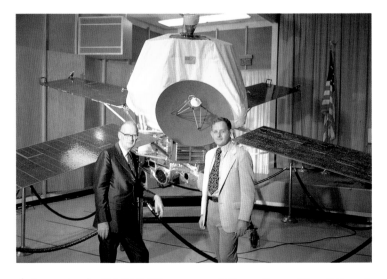

Astronaut–scientist Phil Chapman and the author with a full-scale model of *Mariner* 9 at the Jet Propulsion Laboratory, Pasadena, in November 1971.

Bruce Murray adopted the role of sceptical geologist, making the very good points that 'Lowell's legacy is still plaguing us' and that 'optimism about Mars . . . somehow has extended and endured beyond the realm of science to so grab hold of man's emotions and thoughts that it has actually distorted scientific opinion about it. So it isn't just the popular mind that has been misled, but the scientific mind as well . . . We *want* Mars to be like the Earth.' He went on to say: 'We are all so captive to Edgar Rice Burroughs and Lowell that the observations are going to have to beat us over the head and tell us the answer in spite of ourselves . . .' Well, as Murray confessed later, *Mariner* 9 did indeed 'beat him over the head'.

My own statement paid tribute to Bradbury, Weinbaum and Wells – and to Lowell:

Whatever we can say about his observational abilities, we can't deny his propagandistic power, and I think he deserves credit at least for keeping the idea of planetary astronomy alive and active during a period when perhaps it might have been neglected. He certainly did a lot of harm in some ways, but I think perhaps in the long run the benefits may be greater.

Anyway, I was very moved the other day when I visited the Lowell Observatory for the first time and actually looked through his 24in [61cm] telescope. He's buried right beside it; his tomb is in the shape of the observatory itself. I was distressed to find that his papers had been rather neglected and scattered around. As a result, I have initiated a series of events which may now result in his papers being classified and, hopefully, edited. Whatever nonsense he wrote, I hope that one day we will name something on Mars after him, and I'm sure that he won't be forgotten in this area.*

We are now in a very interesting historic moment with regard to Mars. I'm not going to make any definite predictions because it would be very foolish to go out on a limb, but whatever happens, whatever discoveries are made in the next few days or weeks or months, the frontier of our knowledge is moving inevitably outwards.

It was indeed. *Mariner* 9 was a triumphant success, sending back 7000 images over a period of several months. And they were a revelation. As Bruce Murray put it a year after our symposium:

To me, perhaps the most surprising single aspect of the *Mariner* 9 mission was the discovery of huge volcanic features in the equatorial regions of the hemisphere of the planet that had not been observed by *Mariners* 4, 6 or 7. As these features were first observed through the dust-storm, and only the gigantic calderas at their top were visible, I simply couldn't believe that they were larger than any comparable volcanoes on the Earth. When they emerged fully from the dust, we discovered that Nix Olympica was over 300 miles [in fact, about 600km] in diameter and that the caldera at the crest of the volcanic mountain was larger than the *entire* island of Hawaii that stands above the Pacific Ocean.

*He is not. Crater Lowell, a splendid 200km across, is at 81°W, 52°S. Soon after my visit to the Lowell Observatory, the Institute of Physics microfilmed his papers. My own copy of this microfilm is now in the Library of the Royal Astronomical Society, London.

My own postscript to the *Mariner* 9 encounter said, in part:

It now appears that, by one of those ironies not uncommon in science, the earlier *Mariner* results caused the pendulum to swing too far to the other extreme – away from the hopelessly romantic view of Mars. For the few years from 1965 to 1972 Mars was a cosmic fossil like the Moon – no, not even a fossil, because it could never have known life. The depressing image of a cratered, desiccated wilderness was about as far removed from the Lowell–Burroughs fantasy as it was possible to get.

There were some, undoubtedly, who accepted this new 'revelation' with considerable relief – even glee. Now there would be no further fear of that dreaded cry in the night: 'The Martians are coming! The Martians are coming!' We were comfortably alone in the Solar System, if not the Universe . . .

Well, perhaps we are, but it seems more and more unlikely. The new Mars that has suddenly emerged from the *Mariner* 9 photos, a world of immense canyons and volcanoes and erosion patterns and – dare one say? – dried-up seabeds is a much more active and exciting place than we would have ventured to hope only a few years ago. Lowell and Company may yet have been partly right for the wrong reasons . . .

As the *Mariner* 9 evidence started to accumulate early in 1972, many scientists were literally unable to believe their eyes. Mars has the most spectacular scenery ever discovered. Take for example the Valles Marineris, so-named for *Mariner* 9. Think of the Grand Canyon, then quadruple its depth and multiply its average width five times, to an incredible 120km, and finally imagine that it spans the whole North American continent from Los Angeles to New York. Such is the scale of the canyon carved along the Martian equator.

Yet even this is not the planet's most awesome feature, for Mars is dominated by volcanoes that dwarf any on Earth. Nineteenth-century astronomers, peering at the tiny and often blurred image of Mars, noted a bright spot which they had given the astonishingly prescient name Nix Olympica – 'The Snows of Olympus'. Now that the real nature of this marking is known, the name has been changed to Olympus Mons – 'Mount Olympus'. Though most of its brilliance is due to cloud cover, there can be little doubt that there *is* snow on that awesome summit – albeit snow of carbon dioxide, not water. The mightiest of all the Martian volcanoes, Olympus Mons, is

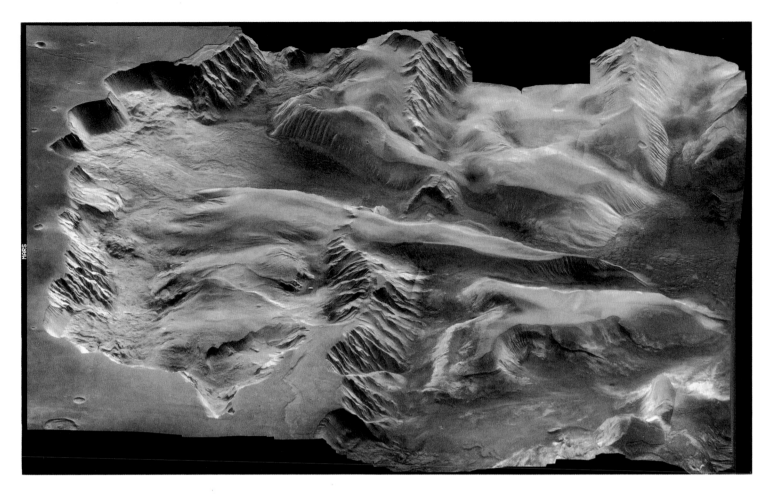

almost three times the height of Everest and about 600km across. Those volcanoes are slumbering now, but not so very long ago, in cosmic terms, they were blasting into the thin atmosphere all the chemicals of life, including water: there are dried-up river beds that give clear indication of recent flash-floods – the first evidence ever found for running water outside our Earth.

Although *Mariner* 9 enormously enlarged our knowledge of Mars during its hundreds of orbits of the planet (it is still there, waiting to be brought back to the Smithsonian), many questions would obviously remain unanswered until robots had landed on the surface of the planet. In the *Mars and the Mind of Man* symposium Bruce Murray stated that

the focus of the entire US planetary program is the *Viking* mission to Mars in 1975–6. It is planned to launch two

A computer-enhanced *Viking* orbiter image of the central region (Candor) of the Mariner Valley (Valles Marineris). Vertical distances have been exaggerated by a factor of two. (*Picture courtesy US Geological Survey*)

identical orbiter-plus-lander spacecraft systems, each with a new large rocket, the Titan–3C/Centaur. Each orbiter/lander combination will weigh about 7500 pounds [3400kg], which can be compared with the weight of *Mariner* after launch, 2200 pounds [1000kg; i.e., one tonne]. The primary objective of the *Viking* mission is the direct search for microbial life on Mars.

The USSR had already made four landing attempts without success. The reasons for these failures are still unknown, and may have been partly sheer bad luck. *Mars* 2 and *Mars* 3 had

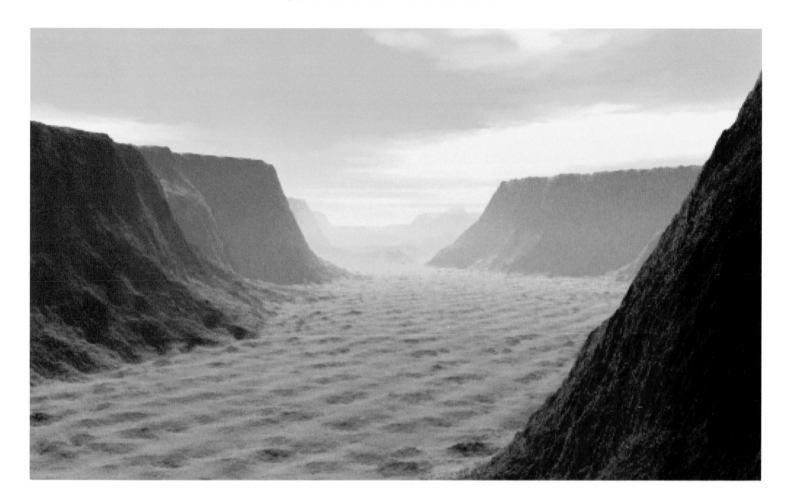

ABOVE: **Rendering by John Hinkley, using Vistapro, of dawn in the Mariner Valley as it might appear now (more accurately, in 1976, the same year as the *Viking* image shown in the previous picture). The mist of water and carbon-dioxide frost which gathered during the night is being slowly dispersed by the rising Sun.** (*Rendering courtesy John Hinkley*)

RIGHT: **One of the most exciting attributes of the Martian surface became increasingly clear as first the *Mariner* and then the *Viking* orbiters revealed to us the features of our neighbour planet: everywhere there were indications that free water had once flowed. Note the 'teardrop' shape of the formation at lower left.** (*Photograph courtesy NASA/JPL*)

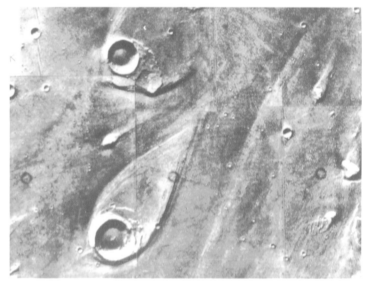

arrived at the height of the great 1971 dust-storm that initially blocked *Mariner* 9's view of the planet; though *Mars* 3 succeeded in landing, it transmitted only twenty seconds of featureless television before signals stopped. *Mars* 6 and 7,

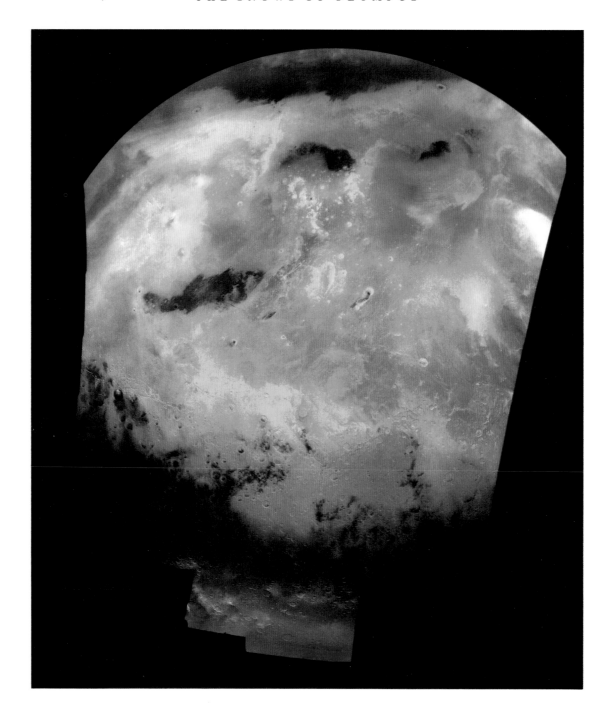

A mosaic of 104 *Viking* orbiter images showing Mars on 11 February 1980; it is centred on the equator at 185°W and extends between 65°N and 65°S. Resolution is better than one kilometre; note the numerous craters and channels (not 'canals'!) in the Southern Hemisphere, and the upper limit of the southern polar icecap, formed of frozen carbon dioxide. The large cloud at the upper right is just to the northwest of Olympus Mons. (*Photograph courtesy US Geological Survey*)

which were launched during the less favourable 1973 'window', did no better. It must have been very disheartening for the scientists involved. (They were equally unlucky a decade later, with the even more elaborate *Phobos* missions.) In striking contrast, the *Vikings* were a triumph for the United States – and specifically for the Jet Propulsion Laboratory (JPL), which designed them, and for their builder, the Hughes Aircraft Company.

Although the *Viking* orbiters mapped the planet with a resolution of 250m, and even ten metres in selected areas, Mars would, as we have said, not become a real place until a camera had gone down to the surface and taken a panoramic view. This is precisely what happened when *Viking* 1 soft-landed on 20 July 1976 (just missing the United States' Bicentennial, owing to an unexpectedly long search for an acceptable landing site), and *Viking* 2 made an equally good touchdown a few weeks later, on 3 September. Both showed panoramic views of a reddish, rock-covered desert, and both collected soil samples for analysis. The atmosphere – about one-hundredth of the density of Earth's – was ninety-seven per cent carbon dioxide, with only a trace of oxygen.

I wonder if any of the scientists and engineers at the Jet Propulsion Laboratory recalled H. G. Wells' story 'The Crystal Egg' (1897) as they waited for the images from the *Viking* lander to appear, line by line, on their monitors. It was surely one of the great moments in the history of space exploration when human eyes first looked across the Plain of Gold (or Planitia Chryse, where *Viking* 1 had landed) – even if there were no Martians there to greet them.

In fact, only a very slothful Martian would have been revealed by the *Viking* camera, which took several minutes to scan a single image and transmit it back to Earth. The scene revealed, though historic, was hardly spectacular: only one detail suggested that this was the first view of an alien planet. The sky, which everyone had expected to be a very deep blue, was actually salmon-pink, owing to the presence of wind-borne dust particles.

In 'The Crystal Egg' (1897) Wells imagined a similar but more exciting scenario. A London antique dealer had acquired a 'mass of crystal, worked into the shape of an egg and brilliantly polished'. Peering into it under certain conditions of lighting, the astonished owner had a view of a

wide and peculiar countryside . . . he seemed always to be looking at it from a considerable height, as if from a tower or

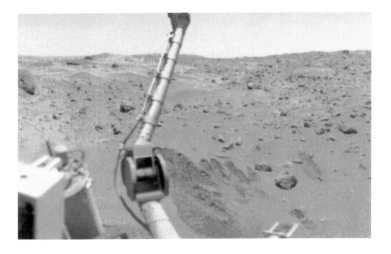

Photograph from the first *Viking* lander, taken on 8 August 1978, two (Earth) years after touchdown. The horizon is a few kilometres away, and most of the rocks in the foreground are about half a metre across. To the right of the arm holding aloft meteorological instruments are the trenches dug by the soil sampler during the (unsuccessful) life-detection experiment. However, if you look carefully you can see the strikingly human-seeming face on the rock immediately above the arm's 'elbow'. It is quite as convincing as the infamous formation in Cydonia (see page 19). (*Photograph courtesy NASA/JPL*)

a mast. To the east and west the plain was bounded at a remote distance by vast reddish cliffs . . . receding in an almost illimitable perspective and fading into the mists . . . There were also trees curious in shape, and in colouring, a deep mossy green and an exquisite grey, beside a wide and shining canal . . .

Needless to say the crystal egg – irretrievably lost, alas, at the end of the story – was somehow relaying images from Mars. This was proved by the fact that there were '*two small moons!* [Wells' italics], one of which moved so rapidly that its motion was clearly visible . . . These moons were never high in the sky, but vanished as they rose; that is, every time they revolved they were eclipsed because they were so near their primary.'

Though they too possessed tentacles, the Martians of 'The Crystal Egg' were far more attractive than the octopoid monsters of *The War of the Worlds* (1898). They were graceful, winged creatures, inhabiting 'splendid buildings, richly coloured and glittering with metallic tracery and facets, among a forest of moss-like and lichenous trees'. Occasionally they peered into the crystal's transmit-receive twin on Mars, and the terrestrial observer was startled when 'the upper part of a face with very large eyes came as it were close to his own'. In addition to several types of aerial Martians there were 'certain broad creatures, in form like beetles but enormously larger' as well as 'clumsy bipeds, dimly suggestive of apes'. And one, 'a vast thing . . . like some gigantic insect, appeared advancing along the causeway beside the canal with extraordinary rapidity. As it drew nearer he perceived that it was a mechanism of shining metals and extraordinary complexity.'

The first question we would have wanted to ask of anything that had crawled, hopped, burrowed or walked within range of *Viking* might appear simple-minded. Whether it had had three heads or four eyes or six tentacles, we would still have wanted to know of any passing Martian: 'Are you identical with us?'

One of the most profound discoveries of the past generation is that, despite all appearances, there is in a sense only a single lifeform on the planet Earth: 'We men, we microbes, we cabbages, we sharks . . .', to paraphrase Carl Sagan. The infinite diversity of the living world is an illusion. Deep down, we are all variations of the same very few biochemical themes. It is as if every creature on Earth were built from one huge organic Meccano set, with only a few basic components. It would be impossible to tell, purely from the disassembled fragments, what any original model was like. So the great unanswered question is this: Must all life, everywhere, depend on the same handful of reactions as it does on Earth? Had we found that Martian lifeforms had just the same chemical themes as terrestrial lifeforms, that would have suggested that no other arrangement is possible. If, on the other hand, it had turned out that Martian life had a fundamentally different chemistry, that would have opened up whole new vistas in biology and, ultimately, medicine. Remember how many of the drugs in the modern pharmacopoeia were discovered by travellers to strange places on our own planet; on a much more sophisticated level, this situation may be repeated in space.

But not on Mars. There is, however, one thing that we science-fiction writers got right: the sands of Mars, shaped by the winds of time into dunes strikingly similar to those found in the deserts of Earth. It may seem surprising that so thin an atmosphere could be so effective, but what the Martian winds lack in mass they make up for in speed.

The two *Viking* landers surveyed their surroundings for a complete Martian year, and in all that time the only local change they observed was a thin layer of frost (probably water and carbon dioxide) on some nearby rocks. However, they also made thousands of temperature and wind-velocity measurements, and collected samples of the local soil to be analysed in the amazingly compact onboard chemical laboratory. After an initial flurry of excitement, however, the hope that organic compounds, perhaps even microorganisms, would be found – the last legacy of Percival Lowell – was disappointed: the Martian soil appeared to be completely sterile, and to contain only traces of the carbon, hydrogen and other elements essential for life ('as we know it', of course; and we probably do not know very much). At both sites the major constituents were silicon and aluminium oxides (i.e., sand) and iron oxides (more familiar as rust, and doubtless responsible for the planet's reddish colour). There is plenty of oxygen on Mars – but it is all locked up in the ground, which is where it would be on Earth if plants did not continually replenish it for the benefit of animal parasites such as us.

The two landing sites had been deliberately chosen to be as safe as possible, and so may well have been in the most uninteresting places on Mars – just as Fate had decreed that *Mariner* would survey the planet's most boring ten per cent. As the *Viking* orbiters had shown, the planet is not all rose-red desert, half as old as Time; it exhibits as much geological variety as Earth, though obviously such life-created formations as coal beds, chalk cliffs and oil-fields are (presumably) absent.

My first full-length novel, *The Sands of Mars* (1951), contains the sentence, '*There are no mountains on Mars*' – italicized, to emphasize the point. After the *Mariner* and *Viking* missions, this caused me considerable embarrassment, and in subsequent printings I apologized to readers. Yet now I would like to retract the retraction – at least partially. On Mars there are indeed no mountains as we know them on Earth and on the Moon. There are cliffs and escarpments and plateaux and canyons, but nothing like the Alps, the Andes or the Himalayas. It is misleading to call even Olympus Mons a mountain – it is much too large! Although almost three times the height of Everest, it spans an area 600km across. More accurate, therefore, to call it a bulge or blister on the face of Mars.

Our own planet has a scale model of Olympus Mons – and, as I have been fortunate enough to discover, it is not only much more spectacular from the ground but more dynamic.

Welcome to Hawaii.

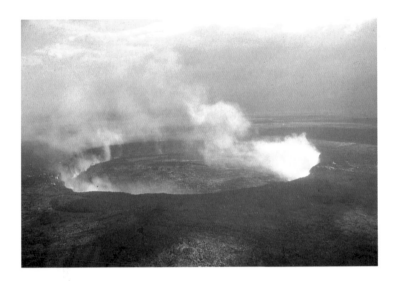

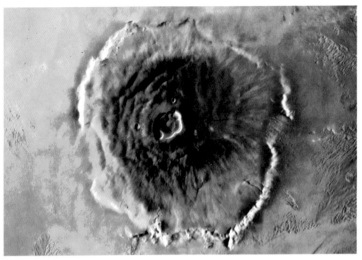

The volcano Kilauea in Hawaii provides a sort of small-scale model of the mighty Olympus Mons. Compare this view across its crater – taken during the author's visit in August 1970 – with the image of the Olympus caldera.

A superb *Viking* orbiter view of Olympus Mons, the greatest mountain in the Solar System. Compare the illustration on page 58. (*Photograph courtesy NASA/JPL*)

In August 1970, at the invitation of Mayor Shunichi Kimura, I toured the Big Island of Hawaii. Among the highlights of the trip were snorkelling off the beach where Captain Cook met his untimely end (a brass plate at the water's edge marks the spot) and visiting the magnificently sited observatory on Mauna Kea, then in an early state of development. In 1970 there was only a cinder road and no power line, so the astronomers had to devote much of their time and energy trucking up drums of diesel fuel from Hilo.

But the most unforgettable incident was my very first helicopter flight, made even more memorable by the fact that it was over an active volcano. Streams of lava were pouring out of Kilauea and had trapped a group of Park Rangers fighting the fires that had been ignited. The Rangers could not have been in any great danger, or passengers such as myself would hardly have been allowed on the 'rescue' mission. Nevertheless, I was much impressed by the sight of an abandoned car on the mountain road – trapped by lava-flows before *and* behind.

Only a few years later I would learn about a volcano which could swallow Kilauea without a hiccup, Olympus Mons. Nevertheless, the Kilauea caldera on Hawaii is extremely instructive – as an approximately 1:10 scale model of its Martian counterpart. Compare the plates above – and then multiply the size of the left-hand caldera by ten.

Another sight that made my flight over Kilauea particularly memorable was of a river of red-hot lava flowing – just beneath our helicopter! – on its way to the sea. Though it was bringing death now, as it burned up the forest on the slopes of the mountain, it was also bringing life. In a few centuries, that chemical-rich lava-flow will be prime Hawaiian farmland. I cannot help wondering if the great Martian volcanoes – Olympus, Arsia, Pavonis and Ascraeus – also helped bring life to their planet, perhaps long before it arose on Earth.

A dozen years after my first visit, another link was forged in the Hawaii–Mars connection, when I met that remarkable man, the late US Senator (and Japanese–US war hero) Spark Matsunaga. Most members of Congress are – understandably – so involved in the day-to-day problems of their constituency that they have little time or energy for the wider view. Not so Spark. A decade after the *Viking* missions he published a remarkable book: *The Mars Project: Journeys Beyond the Cold War* (1986). At a time when such ideas were not popular, it was an eloquent appeal for US–USSR cooperation in space – and, specifically, for a joint mission to Mars.

The year before, on 21 January 1985, he had made this appeal in an almost empty chamber: two Republicans, three Democrats and two dozen spectators. Fortunately the *Congressional Record* carried his words to a wider audience. He opened with a rhetorical question:

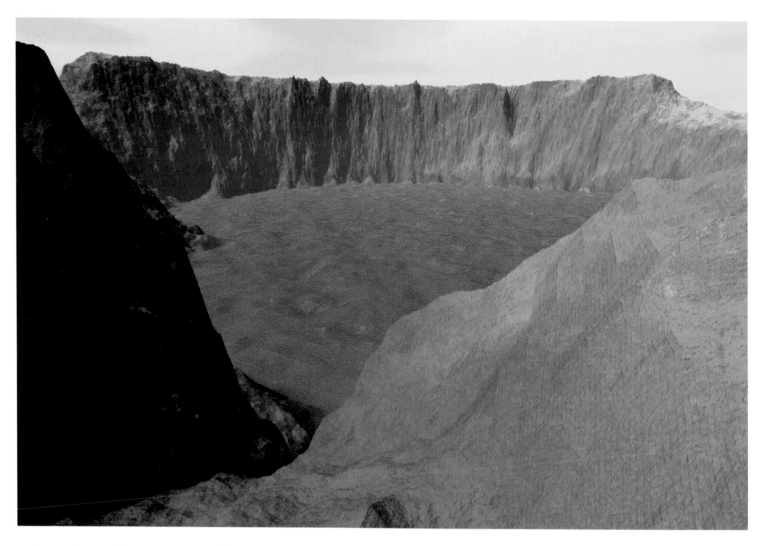

Some of my colleagues may wonder: Has the Senator from Hawaii lost his senses? Here the United States Senate convenes to address a veritable avalanche of pressing issues . . . and the Senator from Hawaii talks about Mars? But, Mr President, I believe we also have a duty to see beyond the cascading issues that engulf us daily . . .

Senator Matsunaga had first become actively interested in space in 1980, when he had visited the newly established observatory complex on Mauna Kea, more than four kilometres above sea-level. As he wrote later:

Memories of that visit to the summit of Mauna Kea have never been far from my thoughts. They stand in sharp

Arsia Mons in the year 100,000,000BC – a Vistapro rendering by John Hinkley. The date may be incorrect by one zero, but not two! This view of the central caldera of the southernmost of the three Tharsis volcanoes – Arsia, Pavonis and Ascraeus – shows how it might have appeared when the lava flood was solidifying. (*Rendering courtesy John Hinkley*)

contrast to the political world I inhabit. I have no illusions about the international scientific community. Like everyone else, scientists are prone to rivalries and petty jealousies. Nevertheless, they still feel the powerful unifying pull of a common language and shared goals. For a practical politician, their unity holds a special appeal.

28

Two years afterwards he became alarmed by the increasing volume of speculation about an arms race in outer space. He was perhaps one of the first to point out that, if the United States and the USSR did engage in such a suicidal diversion of their scientific and industrial manpower, the winner of the Cold War would be . . . Japan, whose industrial resources would not be thus wastefully dissipated. So he started a campaign, in and out of Congress, to promote cooperation rather than conflict. 'Only space,' he wrote, 'offers an arena, a theme, and an organizing principle grand enough to liberate us from the closed loop of insanity that has ensnared us.'

He was surprised to discover that there had already been much more US–USSR cooperation on the scientific level than was generally realized. Moreover, it had not – as some critics alleged – been a one-way affair. The United States had gained as much as the USSR – in some cases, perhaps more. The *Apollo–Soyuz* rendezvous of 1975, though largely symbolic, had been the highpoint of *detente* in space. There had been ambitious plans to follow it up with, among other things, a Shuttle mission to the *Salyut* space station, and indeed an agreement to this effect was signed in May 1977. Then the Cold War hotted up again, largely as a result of the USSR's behaviour towards Poland, and the United States cancelled the whole project. Matsunaga entitled his chapter on this episode 'A Great Lost Opportunity'.

In 1984 he felt it was time to make a new effort, and he approached Carl Sagan, Isaac Asimov and James Michener (who had in 1982 published his novel *Space*) to support a Joint Resolution (SJ 236), 'Relating to cooperative East–West ventures in space'. Needless to say, all three responded enthusiastically – as did I, when he approached me shortly afterwards. Although the fact that I lived halfway around the world precluded my attending in person, I sent him a presentation on videotape.* Alas, the Committee never saw it, although the transcript was put into the record. The rules forbade viewing videotaped testimony, on the grounds that too many witnesses would avoid direct questioning by sending in tapes – a much neater ploy than taking the notorious Fifth Amendment. Nevertheless, I am very happy that my 'virtual presence' helped strengthen Matsunaga's hand.

As he was finishing his plea for joint East–West cooperation that might 'contribute to an international manned mission to Mars, perhaps at the turn of the century', something unexpected happened. Senator William Proxmire entered the chamber and listened intently. Famous (or infamous) for his Golden Fleece Awards for what he considered wasteful research projects, the Senator had long been one of NASA's severest critics. A particular target for his ironic wit had been the proposed SETI (Search for Extra-terrestrial Intelligence) program. He had suggested, not unreasonably, that the money would be better spent on a search for intelligent life in Washington . . . So Senator Matsunaga was somewhat alarmed at this addition to his small but select audience. Great was his relief when Proxmire not only asked permission to co-sponsor the resolution, but added, 'I want to congratulate the Senator from Hawaii on this resolution, an excellent resolution . . .'

In its final form, the resolution was signed by President Reagan on 30 October 1984. It was a fairly mild and non-controversial document, seeking to 'initiate talks with the Government of the Soviet Union, and with other governments . . . for cooperative ventures in such areas as space medicine and space biology, planetary science, manned and unmanned space exploration'. It did *not* contain any specific reference to Mars; hence Senator Matsunaga put forward a later resolution, SR 46 of 21 January 1985.

Things were by then beginning to move. 1985 happened to be the tenth anniversary of the *Apollo–Soyuz* rendezvous, and the two crews had a warm reunion in Washington. Matsunaga took this opportunity to introduce another far-sighted resolution, SR 177 (17 July 1985), 'Relating to an International Space Year'. This followed up my suggestion that 1992 – the quincentennial of Columbus' voyage – would be an appropriate time to start planning an international Mars mission.

Tragically, Spark Matsunaga did not live to see the outcome of his heroic endeavours: he died on 15 April 1990. Though I met him in person only once (during my last visit to Hawaii, in 1984), it is a privilege to have known him.

---

*Senator Matsunaga's description of his dealings with me, including a transcript of my presentation, forms Appendix 1, page 105.

3
Going There

The first flight to the Moon was a major theme of science fiction up to the 1960s. It had a long run for its money – almost two millennia if such fantasies as Lucian's *True History* (*c.*AD150) are accepted, and three centuries if Johannes Kepler's *Somnium* (1634) is taken as the earliest attempt at a realistic portrayal of lunar conditions. The 'first voyage to Mars' tale, by contrast, will have a much briefer career, and its end is already in sight. Perhaps for this reason, there now seems to be a minor boom in such stories: before discussing the realities of a Mars mission I would like to mention three outstanding recent fictional accounts, while apologizing to the authors I have neglected.

Mission to Mars (1990) by *Apollo* 11 Command Module pilot Michael Collins is noteworthy in part because of the author's own space missions, including the most historic of all. The fact that Collins is an excellent writer also does no harm. A skilful combination of fact and fiction, *Mission to Mars* describes an internationally crewed flight that would leave Earth on 3 June 2004 and return twenty-two months later after a forty-day stay on Mars. Only chemical propellants would be used, but fuel requirements would be reduced by making a close approach to Venus and thus getting a boost from the planet's gravitational field. In the course of the novel Collins makes an eloquent plea for the establishment of a permanent Mars base, ultimately leading to a colony.

Ben Bova's *Mars* (1992) is pure fiction, but the scientific and technical details are as carefully worked out as in Collins' book – as one would expect from a veteran science-fact and -fiction author and a past editor of the longest-running magazine in the field, *Analog*. Without sacrificing plausibility, Bova maintains excitement while neatly leaving open the question of life on Mars – past or present.

The final book, Jack Williamson's *Beachhead* (1992), is one in which I must confess an interest: I wrote a preface to it, in gratitude for the many hours of pleasure and inspiration that its author has given me over the years. In this book Williamson takes on the same challenge as Bova – seeing if it would be possible to write an exciting story about the pioneering Mars expedition without inventing details which might be refuted in a few years' time.

I had the uncanny experience of reading *Beachhead* while generating the pictures in this book. Since it requires thirty minutes or more for a high-resolution image to build up on the screen, I read Williamson's manuscript while waiting for the computer to finish its run. And because for obvious reasons we had both chosen the most spectacular areas of Mars, I was reading about such places as the Coprates Canyon and Olympus Mons *while they were slowly materializing on the monitor beside me!*

Interplanetary travel involves concepts which are unfamiliar – and may even seem paradoxical – to creatures adapted to terrestrial conditions. Space is a much simpler environment than that on the surface of any world – especially one like Earth, with its complex geography and meteorology.

All the types of movement we are accustomed to are controlled by two powerful and relentless forces, never absent for a moment: friction and gravity. Friction quickly brings all terrestrial motion – whether it be on land or sea or in the air – to a halt. The nearest we get to frictionless movement on Earth is ice-skating; even here, a gentle application of force is necessary to maintain speed. And at high velocities, in *any* terrestrial medium, enormous amounts of power are required to overcome resistance; hence the jet engine.

In space, on the other hand, there is so little friction that it can be discounted entirely; as Sir Isaac Newton first pointed out, this is why the orbiting Moon has not long ago fallen down to Earth. A spacecraft given any initial velocity will maintain the same speed forever . . . unless accelerated or slowed down by the gravitational field of a nearby celestial body.

The controlling gravitational field in the Solar System is that of the Sun, which keeps all the planets, comets, asteroids, cosmic junk and space-probes moving in highly predictable orbits. We are not aware of its effect here on the Earth's surface, because we are immersed in our own planet's gravitational field, which is – locally – hundreds of times greater, although the solar field is still powerful enough to influence tides in the oceans and atmosphere.

The problem of getting from one planet to another therefore involves climbing out of one intense but localized gravitational field, moving up or down the far more extended field of the Sun, and then descending into another planet's field without acquiring a dangerous terminal velocity. The energy – and hence amount of propellant – required for any particular journey is not proportional to the actual *distance* travelled: all that matters are the various gravity fields involved.

Space travel is rather like a game of cosmic billiards, played on an enormous and frictionless table. To make the game really difficult, the table is not flat, and the 'pockets' are all of different depths, very far apart and moving at high velocities. The challenge is to get out of one pocket and into another, using the minimum amount of energy.

The basic mathematics of space travel was worked out a century ago by the Russian schoolmaster Konstantin Tsiolkovsky and elaborated by later theoreticians and practical engineers, of whom the best-known were Robert Goddard (United States), Hermann Oberth (Romania/Germany), Wernher von Braun (Germany/United States) and Sergei Korolev (USSR). Few people took them seriously until the closing months of World War II, when the V2 rocket proved that, for better *and* for worse, a revolutionary new method of propulsion had arrived – and one which, unlike all others, could operate in the empty void beyond the Earth.

Science-fiction writers had, of course, known this for years. Jules Verne had used rockets in his classic *From the Earth to the Moon* (1865), although only for steering; his astronauts relied on an impossible 'space-gun' to shoot them into space. For the next half century, few authors ventured beyond the Moon: a notable exception being John Jacob Astor, whose *A Journey in Other Worlds* (1894) covered much of the Solar System; his spaceship, like H. G. Wells' in *The First Men in the Moon* (1901), depended on antigravity – which, at least in such a naïve form, is impossible.

The first account of a journey to Mars that was not pure fantasy but had some technical basis was probably the novella 'The Voyage of the *Asteroid*' and its sequel 'The Wreck of the *Asteroid*' (*Wonder Stories*, 1932) by Laurence Manning, an active member of the American Rocket Society and thus familiar with the latest researches in the still infant science of astronautics. An unusually far-sighted visionary (even for a science-fiction writer!), Manning is best remembered for his *The Man Who Awoke* series, much of which is even more relevant now than when it was written, more than half a century ago. In one episode the people of AD5000 castigate our 'false civilization of waste' for exhausting the world's coal and petroleum supplies; in another, humanity is enslaved by a computer; and in 'The City of Sleep' our descendants in AD15,000 spend their entire lives wired into dream-inducing machines. I cannot help fearing that Manning's anticipation of virtual reality may arrive about 13,000 years sooner than he imagined . . .

But back to Mars. Manning's spaceship *Asteroid* first touches down on the inner moon, Phobos; and here Manning made a very curious – and instructive – mistake. (He may have done it for the sake of dramatic effect.) The intrepid explorers are bounding across the face of the tiny world in a gravity field about a thousandth that of Earth's. Overhead, the huge red-and-ochre disc of Mars – more than *five hundred* times the apparent area of our full Moon! – dominates the sky. In his understandable exuberance an astronaut jumps a little too vigorously – and exceeds Phobos' minuscule escape velocity. He continues to fall *upwards*, towards the looming face of Mars. His companions have to make a hurried take-off to rescue the careless high-jumper before the gravity of Mars seizes him.

In fact, the only danger our hero had to worry about was running out of oxygen: there was not the slightest chance that he would add a new crater to the Martian landscape. Even granted that he could jump off Phobos,* he would still possess its full orbital velocity of 7700kph, and would merely become another satellite of Mars, moving in an orbit imperceptibly different from that of Phobos itself. In fact, after half a revolution (just under four hours) the two orbits would intersect and he would return to his starting point, moving at exactly the speed with which he had left it.

Only ten years after the *Asteroid* saga was published the first

---

*Not possible, especially for a man wearing a spacesuit: the potato-shaped satellite's dimensions – 28km × 22km × 18km – make it slightly too large for such a feat. Astronauts might have better luck on the outer moon, Deimos (16km × 12km × 10km).

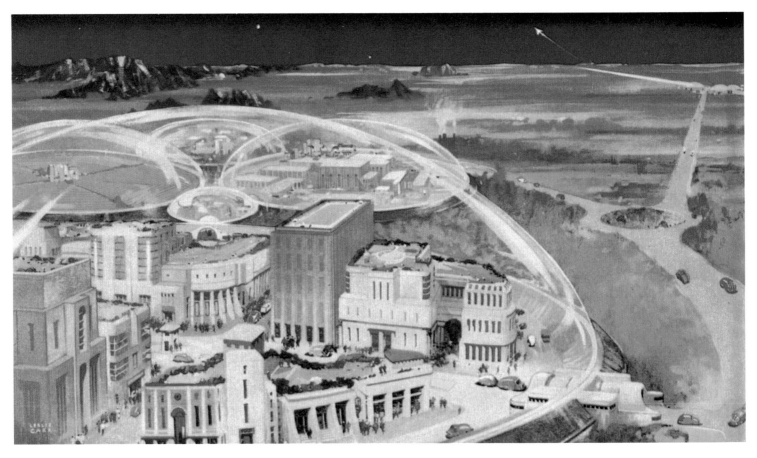

rocket left the Earth's atmosphere when the German V2 (A4) missile made a successful test flight on 3 October 1942. And just ten years after *that* the engineer who had run the secret rocket program at Peenemunde, Wernher von Braun, published an extensive technical analysis which showed that an expedition to Mars would be possible – even using existing knowledge and conventional fuels. His *The Mars Project* (originally published in German in 1952; English-language editions 1953, 1991) may be regarded as a thought experiment. He did not really expect that we would go to Mars with the relatively primitive technology and propellants of the 1950s, but he wanted to prove that it *could* be done, even making the most conservative assumptions. It was as if the Wright brothers, immediately after the first heavier-than-air flight at Kitty Hawk in 1903, had begun to draw up plans for transatlantic crossings.

Von Braun argued that a Mars Mission should not be entrusted to a single vessel (pointing out that Columbus, very wisely, used three). He proposed a flotilla of no less than ten

Artists' 'preconstructions' of how a Martian base might look a couple of centuries hence. This painting by Temple Press house artist Leslie Carr, based on a drawing by R. A. Smith, was made for my book *The Exploration of Space* (1951). Note the surface vehicles (Marswagons) leaving through the airlock, the use of multiple domes for safety, and the farm area (part of the air-purification setup) at top left. Arizona's controversial Biosphere II experiment (see page 44) is the first attempt to model such a system here on Earth. More details of how a base like this might function are given in my 1951 novel *The Sands of Mars*.

spaceships, each with a seven-person crew. These would be assembled and fuelled in Earth orbit, and would have a mass of 3720 tons *each*. Though this must have seemed an enormous figure at a time when the world's largest rocket weighed fifteen tons, it is almost the same as that of the Saturn-V which carried the first men to the Moon just two decades later. However,

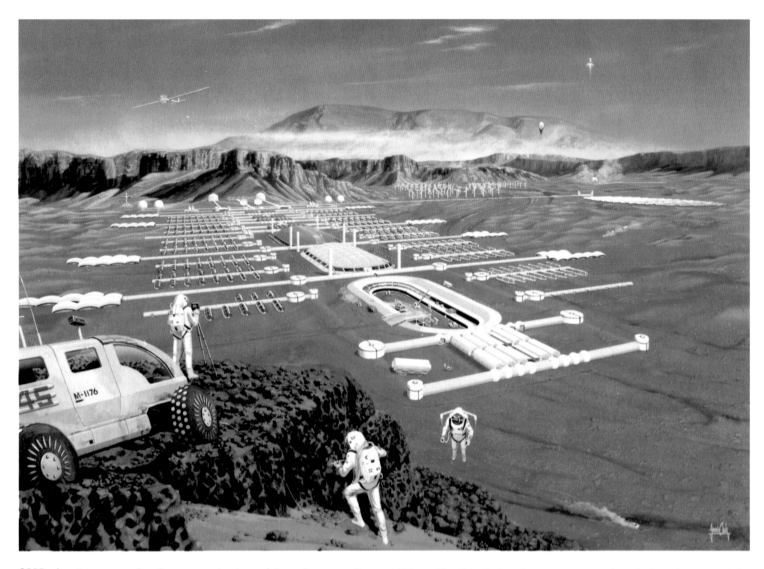

3000-plus tons was the Saturn rocket's weight *when standing on the launchpad*; the payload it could deliver to LEO (Low Earth Orbit) was only 150 tons. Von Braun's 3720-tonners would start with that mass *from orbit* on their 260-day voyage to Mars.

To assemble and supply them would require a fleet of forty-six three-stage ferries or space shuttles, each weighing 6400 tons at take-off and capable of lifting thirty-nine tons to orbit: this is twice the capacity of the US Shuttle, but less than half that of the Russian *Energia*, the only heavy-lift vehicle currently in existence. These ferries would have to make almost 1000 flights, burning five million tons of fuel, before the Mars flotilla would

Where Carr's painting (OPPOSITE) was done before the start of the Space Age, this Japanese view (by an unnamed artist) was executed in the 1990s, and is correspondingly hi-tech in its expectations. Yet similar problems have in fact been solved in similar ways. The farming area has been split up to form numerous separate sections (the 'flanges' of the structures resembling television aerials to either side of the central axis), while residential areas are for safety segregated into several domes set at a distance from the main complex. (*Painting reproduced by permission of Obayashi Corporation*)

be ready to break loose from the Earth's gravitational field.

Once the ten spaceships had gone into orbit around Mars, fifty of the astronauts would go down to the surface in three 'landing boats' and spend 449 days exploring the planet. (A much shorter time would certainly be preferable, but this long 'waiting period' is necessary for Earth and Mars to get into the right positions for the minimum-energy return journey.) Altogether, the mission would last slightly less than three years – as did the first circumnavigation of our own planet (20 September 1519 to 8 September 1522); however, unlike Magellan's crew, of whom over ninety per cent, including the commander, died *en route*, the voyagers to Mars would be in constant touch with home. The psychological importance of this could be enormous – even decisive.

Von Braun estimated the total cost of his Mars Project would be about that of 'a minor military operation extending over a limited theatre of war'. An interesting comparison, but also a depressing one, since it is hard to imagine that even a peaceful world society would allocate such funding for a purely scientific project. Fortunately, as von Braun pointed out in the 1962 revision of his book, developments in rocket engineering had made his earlier calculations much too pessimistic. He was happy to retract his comparison, asserting that 'on the basis of technological advancements available or in sight in the year 1962, a large expedition to Mars will be possible in fifteen or twenty years at a cost which will be only a minute fraction of our yearly national defense budget'.

The main 'technological advancement' was the mastery of cryogenic (low-temperature) propellants, particularly liquid hydrogen. The 1952 edition of *The Mars Project* had assumed that, especially for missions lasting several years, it would be necessary to use propellants which remained liquid at room temperatures; von Braun had chosen the combination of hydrazine (N_2H_4) and nitric acid. Because the performance of a rocket depends exponentially on the velocity of its exhaust gases, the fifty per cent increase provided by a liquid hydrogen–oxygen combination would put *five* times as much payload in orbit for a *quarter* of the originally planned take-off weight! The Mars Project need no longer cost as much as a small war; more like a border skirmish . . .

To return to the analogy of heavier-than-air flight, the line of engineering development from the Wright biplane to the DC3 – even the DC6 – did not involve any revolutionary new inventions. Almost every feature of propeller-driven aircraft up to the 1950s was there, in embryo, in the 1903 'Flyer', but innumerable refinements had multiplied efficiency to improve performance out of all recognition. In the same way, there is no doubt that conventional chemical rockets of the type perfected by von Braun and his opposite number in the USSR, Sergei Korolev, could take us to Mars for a fraction of the money now being made available by the ending of the Cold War.

Numerous paper studies of Mars Missions have been made by NASA and other space-orientated organizations. One of the most recent and most impressive is the *Mars Mission Final Report*, published by the International Space University (ISU) after its fourth annual session in Toulouse, France, in August 1991. During their ten-week residency 137 students from twenty-six countries took intensive courses in every aspect of space studies – engineering, political, medical, legal and economic. Yet, virtually in their spare time, they managed to compile a 600-page volume rivalling anything that could be produced by governmental or industrial organizations – and, I suspect, with a much higher percentage of novel ideas.

The report envisages an International Mars Mission (IMM) far less ambitious in scale (and cost) than that imagined by von Braun almost half a century earlier. However, thanks to huge advances in rocket engineering and in robotics, it could be a much more effective one. It would be divided into three phases – precursor, cargo and piloted – with the first two being entirely automatic, and with humans travelling only on the last.

In the precursor mission, targeted for 2003–14, robot probes would be sent to locate suitable landing sites and resources. These advance scouts – successors to *Mariner* and *Viking* – would include rovers and several thousand 'microrobots' weighing only about fifty grams (two ounces!) each. These mechanical insects would be scattered over large areas, and would radio back their observations to mother robots, and hence to Earth *via* relay satellites in orbit. If this scenario appears somewhat fantastic, bear in mind that all the necessary microminiaturization technology already exists, and should have reached the required degree of maturity by then.

When the precursor mission had been completed and a landing site selected as a result of its observations, an automatic space-freighter would be launched (target date 2014) on a 'cargo mission' to Mars carrying the supplies and equipment the Marsnauts would need on their arrival, in 2016.

The first manned expedition would stay only forty days but would lay the groundwork (and leave much of the equipment) for a 400-day mission starting in 2018. Each mission would have a crew of eight travelling in a single vehicle – unlike von Braun's seventy in a flotilla of ten – and, instead of needing hundreds of ferry flights by 6000-ton monsters to assemble and provision the Mars ship in orbit, the IMM (International Mars Mission) scenario would require only nineteen flights by a vehicle which is already in existence, the Russian *Energia*. This enormous reduction in scale would be made possible by the use of nuclear energy for the Earth–Mars transfer, with chemical propellants being reserved for low-orbit operations around both planets.

Nuclear reactions can provide virtually unlimited amounts of energy at any power level – up to that required to vaporize a city. A large H-bomb can liberate enough gigawatt-centuries to lift a million tons to Mars: but sheer energy cannot, by itself, propel a spacecraft. Some kind of working fluid has to be expelled to provide thrust. Two different routes – thermal and electric – to nuclear propulsion for space vehicles have been successfully demonstrated, though only the latter has been used in actual operations (for such modest tasks as keeping satellites on station).

The nuclear-thermal (not to be confused with thermonuclear!) rocket (NTR) is basically the same as the conventional liquid-propellant rocket, except that the working fluid – usually hydrogen – is heated by a nuclear instead of a chemical reaction before it expands through the nozzle to produce thrust. In a series of classic papers published more than forty years ago in the *Journal of the British Interplanetary Society*,* L. R. Shepherd and A. V. Cleaver showed the advantages of such a system, and described how it might be realized in practice by using a uranium reactor operating at very high temperature. Such an 'atomic rocket' is attractive because hydrogen is the ideal working fluid, giving several times the exhaust velocity of the best chemical propellants.

Between 1955 and 1973 the US Atomic Energy Commission and the US Air Force spent a billion and a half dollars on the NERVA program, whose ground-tests demonstrated that uranium-fission reactors could power rockets much more effi-

*'The Atomic Rocket', *JBIS*, September and November 1948, January and March 1949. A non-technical description of such a rocket, based on the paper by Shepherd and Cleaver, appears in my novel *Prelude to Space* (1951).

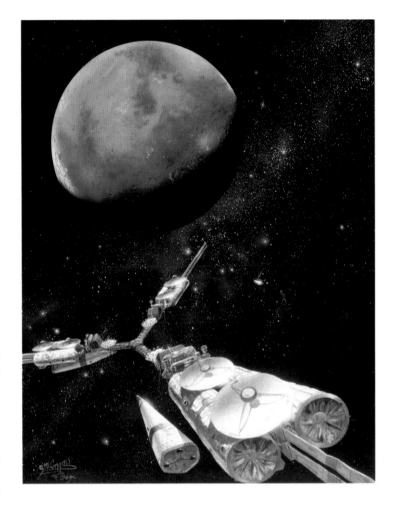

A new wave of colonists from Earth approaches Mars aboard one of the cumbersome vessels used for ferrying people and vital supplies between the two planets. Such spaceships, of course, require no streamlining or other features designed to cope with an atmosphere, for space is their only habitat: built there, they will never touch down on a planet. (*Painting by Michael Carroll, reproduced by permission*)

ciently than chemical energy. However, the effort was then abandoned because there appeared to be no operational requirement for a nuclear rocket. In any event, for reasons which are much clearer now than in the optimistic 1960s, nuclear-thermal rockets are quite unacceptable for lift-offs from Earth, or even for low-orbit operations. Sooner or later there would be a *Challenger*-type disaster, and tons of radioactive material would be dispersed over most of our planet. Nevertheless, NTRs may yet have an important role in deep space – unless they are superseded by something better.*

The alternative, nuclear-electric propulsion (NEP), was chosen for the IMM as being simpler and safer; it would present no danger to the Earth because it can operate only in space. NEP uses electrical fields, not heat, to accelerate charged particles; the hardware is a giant version of the cathode-ray tube whose stream of hurtling electrons brings the world into your living-room. That stream of electrons, when it hits the television screen, produces an infinitesimal recoil. If you took the whole assembly out into space, and opened up the tube so that the electrons could escape, you would have a simple 'electric rocket'; but you would have to wait quite a while before you saw any sign of movement. A practical NEP system (also known as an 'ion thruster') uses not lightweight electrons but heavy atoms such as those of mercury or the noble gas xenon. In fact, any material that can be given a charge so that it reacts to an electric field could be used. This flexibility of NEP may be one of its most important features; being able to extract the propellant for the return to Earth from the Martian atmosphere would completely transform the economics of the IMM scheme. (What would be the price of a transatlantic air ticket today if fuel had to be carried for the return journey?)

The final design for an NEP vessel that would carry a crew of eight to Mars is, I am delighted to say, very similar to *2001*'s spaceship *Discovery* – and for the same engineering reasons. It consists of a long truss (or backbone) with crew quarters at one end and the reactor-propulsion assembly at the other – and even a long-range communications dish poking out near the middle! The vessel would, again like *Discovery*, provide artificial gravity by rotation.

The ISU report estimated that the cost of the project (i.e., precursor and cargo missions, followed by two piloted missions) would be (in 1991 dollars) $239 billion, and that additional missions would cost about $20 billion each. Substantial sums, of course, but very much less than those required for von Braun's version. (By comparison, the cost to the United States alone of the Gulf War was $60 billion and the total bill must have been several times that – more than sufficient for the IMM.)

It seems certain, therefore, that human beings could visit Mars in the early part of the twenty-first century – *if* the resources were made available. The ISU report discusses in some detail the setting up of an 'International Space Exploration Organization' (ISEO) to finance and operate such a mission. Yet is this likely to happen, in a world beset with political, economic and above all environmental problems?

The first landing on the Moon does not provide a good parallel. When the history of the Space Age is written, the *Apollo* program will be seen as a major anomaly caused entirely by political considerations. The decision to go to the Moon was the reaction of the United States (and specifically of President Kennedy) to the series of technological humiliations beginning with *Sputnik* and Gagarin and culminating in the military disaster of the Cuban invasion. It was a product of the Cold War, a chapter of history which has now ended. If there had been no confrontation between the United States and the USSR, and space technology had been driven by purely scientific and commercial considerations, the first landing on the Moon might still be decades in the future.

It is hard – though not impossible – to think of any scenario which would, as *Apollo* did for the Moon, accelerate the course of history so that a Mars mission would occur *as soon as it became technically feasible*. What is more likely is that astronautical knowledge and engineering skills will steadily increase until, at some time in the next century, it becomes clear that a flight to Mars is a reasonable extension of current technology, largely using extant hardware.

A good case can be made for going back to the Moon first, and learning how to live there – only a couple of days' flight-time from the safety of the home planet – before risking the long haul to Mars. The ISU report rejects this argument, concluding:

In summary, we would simply like to state that a lunar base may well be a worthwhile and necessary component of an overall plan in increasing human presence in space. It may in fact be a useful infrastructure element towards the exploration of Mars. But as our mission design evolved, it became more and more evident that a lunar facility was simply not required, and has therefore not been baselined in the IMM.

---

*Early in 1992 the Pentagon revealed that it had so far spent $130 million on a secret 'Space Nuclear Thermal Propulsion' program, and that ground-tests were expected shortly. The Russians, too, have operated an advanced nuclear rocket. They wanted to show it at a US aerospace conference recently, but the customs authorities at Los Angeles Airport would not let them bring their model into the country!

It is true that a diversion of resources to a lunar facility would delay a pioneering Mars mission, and even dilute some of the enthusiasm for it ('We went there *last* year . . .'), but in this case it might be wise to hasten slowly: spending extra time and money on the Moon could save many lives on the road to Mars. This point was made very strongly by Paul D. Lowman of the Goddard Space Flight Center in his paper 'American Space Programs, 1965 to 2019: A Critical Review' (July 1990). I quote: 'It is the author's considered opinion that establishment and operation of a manned lunar outpost is an *absolutely essential prerequisite to an eventual manned Mars program* [author's emphasis].' Lowman argues that establishing a lunar outpost will provide vital operational experience for an eventual Mars mission – far more quickly and at much lower risk and cost. Conditions on the two worlds are similar enough that any equipment or technology developed on the Moon can be easily adapted to Mars.

And, taking the longer-term view, the Moon might play a vital role in the exploration of the Solar System by providing a low-gravity base. It requires less than one-twentieth of the energy to escape from the Moon than from the Earth; when there is a fully established lunar industry (sometime in the twenty-second century?) all deep-space vessels would be built there – or in close orbit – so that, never having to fight their way up through the Earth's massive gravitational field, they could be much more efficiently designed.

There is also the possibility, albeit remote, that deposits of ice may exist on the Moon, either buried or in polar valleys where the Sun never shines and the temperature is always far below zero. Being able to refuel on the Moon would have a major impact on the economics of space travel. In fact, it might not even be necessary to go down to the lunar surface to do this: fuel and cargo could be sent up to lunar orbit. Because the Moon has no atmosphere, it provides an ideal location for realizing the dream, impossible or at least impracticable on Earth, of a 'space-gun'. Many years ago* I suggested the use of lunar launch tracks, like the catapults on aircraft-carriers, to loft payloads into space utilizing electrical energy alone. The velocity needed to attain lunar orbit from the Moon's surface would require a track two kilometres long if it operated at an acceleration of one hundred gees (twenty kilometres at

*'Electromagnetic Launching as a Major Contribution to Space Flight', *Journal of the British Interplanetary Society*, November 1950.

ten gees). Once the considerable capital investment had been made, cargo and propellants could be put into space cheaply by this means.

There are many other ways in which the overall cost of space travel might be reduced. Perhaps the most promising involve more advanced nuclear technology. Uranium (or plutonium) fission is messy and inefficient, and for years the Holy Grail of the atomic engineers has been the achievement of controlled nuclear fusion. The ISU report emphasizes that 'no rocket can compete with a fusion rocket as an interplanetary vehicle', and stresses the importance of the reaction involving deuterium and tritium (two isotopes of hydrogen). A few months after the ISU team published their findings, the scientists working with the Joint European Torus (JET) announced that they had achieved a net energy gain with this reaction. It does look as if hydrogen may be the key to the Universe in ways other than the obvious – first as a chemical propellant to reach space, and thereafter as a nuclear fuel to cross the gulfs between the planets. This may happen sooner than we imagine if the current worldwide research on so-called 'cold' fusion is successful.

Among even more exotic possibilities is the use of antimatter, whose fundamental particles have charges the reverse of normal (to us) matter. If matter and antimatter are brought into contact the result is total annihilation, with the conversion of all the mass involved into pure energy. Add a pinch of antimatter to, say, a large volume of water, and the result would be a rapidly expanding mass of superheated steam which could easily provide rocket propulsion.

It is currently possible to make minute quantities of antimatter in particle accelerators, but only at great expense. Even if it could be manufactured in bulk, how do you handle such an incredibly dangerous material? In theory, it could be done by suitably designed magnetic and electrical fields, and a number of scientists (notably Robert Forward) think this is the way to go – maybe late in the next century.

There is another, much more benign way of crossing space: the solar sail. The pressure of the radiation from the Sun is tiny – at the Earth's distance it amounts to a few millionths of a gram over the area of your hands. But out in space even this tiny pressure can be important, because it is acting all the time, and, unlike rocket fuel, it is free and unlimited. Using materials already in existence, we could build huge, very lightweight sails to catch the radiation blowing from the Sun. The acceleration these sails would give us would be minuscule – about one-thousandth of a gee, perhaps – so that in the first second our sail-powered craft would move only about half a centimetre, but after a minute it would have gone nearly twenty metres and be travelling at nearly two kilometres per hour: not bad for something driven by pure sunlight! After an hour it would be about sixty-five kilometres from the starting-point and moving at 130kph, and at the end of a day's run the velocity would be something like 3000kph; escape velocity would be reached within a couple of days.

If all goes well, the first solar-sail mission will take place in 1994, when an Ariane-4 rocket will launch three small space-craft on a race to the Moon. The sponsors will be the World Space Foundation of South Pasadena, the European Union pour la Promotion de la Propulsion Photonique and the Solar Sail Union of Japan.

But the Moon is only the first objective – a convenient target for an experiment intended to try out the technology of deploying and controlling huge, flimsy sheets of mirror-coated plastic film. As Robert Staehle, the World Space Foundation's President, stated in a recent (November 1991) *Newsletter*:

> From the Moon, our Foundation spacecraft is designed to go to Mars. By so doing, we hope to establish that solar sails can be relied upon to haul heavy cargo in advance of the first human explorers of the Red Planet. Many studies show this to be not only practical, but to offer the potential of saving billions of dollars in transportation costs by substituting abundant sunlight for massive loads of propellant which would otherwise have to be hauled up from Earth.

Solar sailing involves no new technologies – rather, the revival of very ancient ones (for that matter, the rocket itself is at least 1000 years old); perhaps the sunjammers of the Space Age may play the same role between the planets that their precursors once did on the oceans of this world. But quite recently there has appeared another concept – the space eleva-tor – which may make spaceflight no more expensive than ordinary travel on the face of the Earth. Or is it such a new idea? According to *Genesis* 11 *iv*, it occurred to the Babylonians when they said, 'Go to, let us build ourselves a city and a tower, whose top may reach unto heaven . . .' Of course, the Tower of Babel suffered a major malfunction (caused, as usual, by communications problems), but perhaps the time has come to try again.

In 1960 a Russian engineer, Yuri Artsutanov, pointed out that it was theoretically possible to lay a cable between a spot on the equator and a satellite hovering in geostationary orbit directly over that spot (as most of today's Comsats do). Once the initial connection had been made, the cable could be reinforced until it was strong enough to lift useful payloads, providing, in effect, an elevator to space – hence the name. Although rocket propulsion would still be required for the rest of the mission, more than ninety per cent of the effort needed to escape from Earth could be provided by weightless electrical energy instead of tons of rocket propellant. The cost of reaching space would be reduced by a factor of hundreds, if not thousands.

There would be another bonus. Rockets are exciting and spectacular, but they are definitely not friendly to the environ-ment. Would you *really* like to live next door to a busy spaceport?

As the geostationary orbit is 26,000km above the equator, it might seem unlikely that any material would be strong enough to span this gulf; the best steel would snap under its own weight if a length of more than a few hundred kilometres was hung vertically. Nevertheless, both theory and laboratory experi-ments hint at materials which would allow the construction of a space elevator – if the volume of traffic ever justified it.

One such possible material has very recently become the focus of much discussion. Professor Richard Smalley and his colleagues at Rice University, Texas, discovered that sheets of carbon atoms can wrap themselves into microscopic tubes, or nanotubes – close relatives of the fullerenes. These latter were named after Buckminster Fuller (whose geodetic domes are based on the same principle) and represent an entirely new arrangement of carbon atoms; the fullerene that grabbed the popular imagination was C_{60}, shaped like a soccer ball. The nanotubes produced to date are microscopically short – as the name suggests – but, if it proves possible to create them at macroscopic lengths, the resulting fibres would be as strong as anything we could ever hope to make.

What a pity that 'Bucky' missed this amazing discovery, which has greatly added to his posthumous fame. He was kind enough to write the sleeve notes to the recording I made from *The Fountains of Paradise*, and mentioned that over a quarter of a century earlier he had anticipated something very similar to the space elevator:

In 1951, I designed a free floating tensegrity ring-bridge to be installed way out from and around the Earth's equator. Within this 'halo' bridge, the Earth would continue its spinning while the circular bridge would revolve at its own rate. I foresaw Earthian traffic vertically ascending to the bridge, revolving and descending at preferred Earth loci.

The first 'small step' towards the space elevator was made in August 1992, when the astronauts on the Space Shuttle *Atlantis* attempted to lower a payload from the Shuttle bay on a twenty-kilometre tether. Although the experiment was only a partial success (a late change in the flight hardware caused the deployment mechanism to jam), it marked the beginning of a new technology. (I'm pleased to say that the crew of *Atlantis* took a copy of my 1979 novel *The Fountains of Paradise* into space with them and showed it during their in-orbit press conference to explain what their experiment might one day lead to. It was a strange experience to see one of my own books floating around weightlessly!)

The point is worth making that, if a space elevator were too difficult or expensive to construct on Earth, it would be relatively easy on Mars, with only one-third of Earth's gravity and a stationary orbit 17,000km above the equator instead of 26,000km. In *The Fountains of Paradise* I suggested an ideal location: the volcano Pavonis Mons, which is exactly on the Martian equator and whose summit, at twenty-seven kilometres, must be above the great dust-storms which sometimes rage across Mars for weeks at a time.

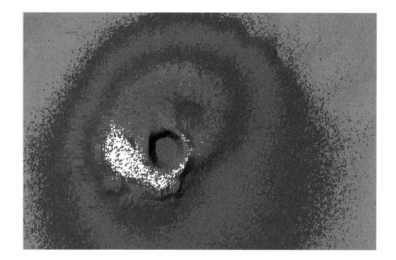

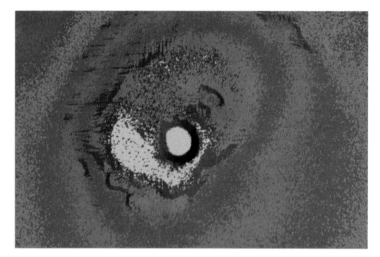

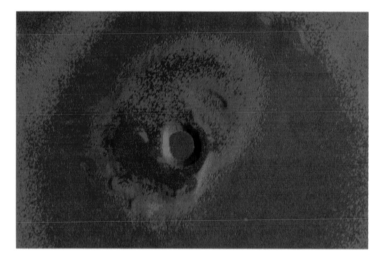

TOP: **The volcano Pavonis Mons as it might appear today from a low-level orbiter. Although this mountain is not as huge as Olympus Mons, it shares – as do Arsia and Ascraeus, the other two of Mars' four great volcanoes – the same height as its larger counterpart: twenty-seven kilometres. It lies exactly on the equator, and for this reason I suggested in *The Fountains of Paradise* (1979) that it would be a good location for the lower terminal of the Martian Space Elevator. In this rendering I have avoided vertical exaggeration and have tried to match the surface coloration with the reality, showing a sprinkling of carbon-dioxide frost. CENTRE: After seven hundred years of terraforming, in AD2700, greenbelting has begun and different species of lichens are spreading at the elevations for which they are best adapted. Some water has accumulated in the caldera, but is still permanently frozen. FOOT: A further century has passed, and now the surrounding plain is completely covered with vegetation – and, for a few weeks at the height of summer, Lake Pavonis thaws out.**

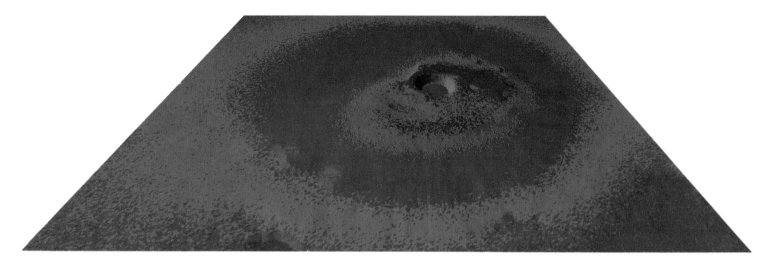

Thanks to the versatility of Vistapro imaging, we don't have to be satisfied with a single view of our projected scene. Here we see the Economy Class tourist's view of Pavonis, approaching the mountain from the south, in the same year, AD2800, as in the previous picture.

There may, however, be one fatal objection to a Martian space elevator – the inner moon Phobos, which orbits the planet at a height of 6000km. Every eight hours this multi-billion-ton body would have a chance of severing the elevator; it might miss on the first few flybys, but sooner or later . . . So we may have to dismantle Phobos – perhaps using it as construction material – or push it up to a higher orbit, like its smaller companion Deimos.

Such feats of astroengineering lie centuries in the future, and are of no practical concern to those planning to visit Mars by ex-President George Bush's optimistic goal of 2019 (see below). But, even if they are regarded as no more than thought experiments, concepts like fusion and antimatter rockets, solar sails, Moon-based launchers and space elevators should remind us of powers and possibilities that remain to be exploited; if we do not use them, it will be because we find something better.

As studies like the ISU report have demonstrated, humans can reach Mars with technologies which already exist. And let us not be too hasty to set limits to what may be done even with these undoubtedly primitive tools. For a beautiful example of such tunnel vision, here is a pronouncement from the US astronomer William Pickering, made while the Wright Brothers were *already* setting new aviation records:

The popular mind often pictures gigantic flying machines speeding across the Atlantic and carrying innumerable passengers in a way analogous to our modern steamships . . . It seems safe to say that such ideas must be wholly visionary, and even if a machine could get across with one or two passengers the expense would be prohibitive to any but the capitalist who could own his own yacht.

Well, the 'popular mind' – can't you hear the professorial sniff? – was completely right, and Pickering had made as big a fool of himself as that other distinguished astronomer, Simon Newcomb, who 'proved' at the turn of the century that heavier-than-air flight was impossible. Pickering's gaffe is what in *Profiles of the Future* (1962) I called a 'failure of nerve'. Even when he wrote those words aircraft were *already* demonstrating the technology that would one day create 'gigantic flying machines . . . carrying hundreds of passengers'. No new invention or discovery was required – merely three or four decades of steady development. And when that had reached its plateau and could go no further, along came the jet engine. When a new technology is really needed, it is always forthcoming.

Pickering was right, however, on one trivial point: there are indeed a few capitalists who have private aerial yachts. What the good professor never imagined was that they would be outnumbered millions to one by economy-class tourists.

But will we ever need the space-going equivalent of today's jumbo jets? Considering the sad fate of once-famous airlines, there is reasonable cause for scepticism. Lunar tourism makes sense, for the Moon is only a couple of days away, and the basic energy cost of a round trip is less than a hundred dollars, assuming a space elevator at both ends. But it takes months to reach Mars by the most economical routes, and few people would be prepared to give up so much of their lives, even if they could afford the fare.

There is another factor, which ours is the first generation to appreciate: it would be impossible to phone home. Even on an Earth–Moon circuit, the three-second time-lag would be annoying. It would be easy to fax your Mars office – but not to *talk* to it.

Yet, if interplanetary cruise times could be reduced from months to weeks, space tourism could become attractive. The ideal case would be if a ship could maintain a steady acceleration of one gee, so that the passengers would feel normal weight for the entire trip (except for ã few minutes at midflight, when the ship had to be turned around to begin decelerating). Rather surprisingly, when the planets are at their closest the one-gee dash from Earth to Mars would take only – two days! The peak velocity at midpoint would be just under a million kph, which is fairly low down the scale of cosmic speeds. Even when they were on opposite sides of the Sun, the constant-acceleration one-gee journey between the two planets would take only a week.

Such feats would require the expenditure of energies *thousands* of times greater than those involved in any missions we could plan today, and might also face other problems, such as the danger of high-speed collision with interplanetary debris. But there is no law of nature that rules them out: if, in the centuries and millennia that lie ahead, our descendants want to reach Mars in a few days, they will be able to do so.

And what about a long weekend there? I think not – at least while we have to rely on rockets or any other *known* form of propulsion: it would be no fun spending the whole trip in a tank of water to withstand the necessary fifty or one hundred gees. Better to wait for shortcuts through hyperspace or radio teleportation – whichever can guarantee that your baggage will arrive before you do, and on the right planet!

I would love to think that Mars brought forth life – perhaps even intelligent life – in the days when it had a thicker atmosphere, running water and a more benign climate. But that is a romantic dream; it is much more probable that, as Ray Bradbury said in a famous short story, *we* will be the First Martians.

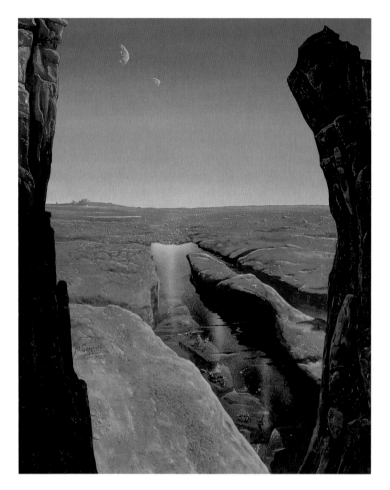

The Last Oasis. **A romantic view by artist Michael Carroll of an early epoch in Mars' great (and still continuing) Ice Age, as the face of the planet at last settles, and the desert triumphs.** (*Painting by Michael Carroll, reproduced by permission*)

There might have been living humans on Mars by this time had it not been for Vietnam, Watergate and other disasters. I still vividly recall Vice-President Spiro Agnew's statement to Walter Cronkite, just thirty minutes after the Saturn-V lift-off on the first mission to the Moon: 'I don't think we'd be out of line in saying we are going to put a man on Mars by the end of the century.'

At that time, such optimism seemed justified; my own short story, 'Transit of Earth' (set in 1984!) is a good example of post-*Apollo* euphoria. During the 1970s NASA study groups hurried to produce reports for Congressional committees describing scenarios that would put humans on Mars before 2000. Today they read like exercises in technological wishful thinking – though perhaps not so remote from reality as those Space-Shuttle studies that predicted weekly flights to orbit, delivering payloads at a tenth of the expendable rockets' price.

On the twentieth anniversary of the *Apollo* landing, President George Bush gave a new target date: 2019, exactly half a century after Armstrong and Aldrin set foot upon the Moon. (As they were both born in 1930, they have a pretty good chance of seeing if the date is met.) Although one hopes that the sort of Cold War confrontation that drove the *Apollo* program will play no future role in human affairs, the date of the Mars landing will probably be determined more by politics and economics than by technology. If for some reason – for example, a challenge by extraterrestrials to prove our fitness to survive! – it were essential to reach Mars without regard to safety or expense, the feat could probably be achieved by the end of the century. However, I doubt if a return trip could be guaranteed, and, even if it was, the astronauts would be facing still largely unknown medical hazards. Although men (as yet, no women) have shown no permanent ill-effects after a full year in space, it seems very probable that artificial gravity may be essential for long-duration flights. There is no fundamental difficulty in providing this, either by spinning the spacecraft or by connecting two sections with a slowly rotating tether; but it would add to complexity, cost and time.

Parallels have often been drawn between space travel and Antarctic exploration, and a quick dash to Mars might well have the same tragic outcome as Scott's ill-fated assault on the South Pole in 1912. Such unnecessary heroics would put back the cause of space exploration by decades. Men did not return to the South Pole for almost half a century after Scott and Amundsen – but, when they did, it was with vastly improved technologies. And this time, they stayed there . . .

In one sense, though, there are *already* people on Mars. As soon as good maps of the planet were available from the *Mariner* and *Viking* missions, the hundreds of newly revealed features had to be given names. This task, traditionally performed by a committee of the International Astronomical Union (IAU), is not an easy one; national emotions and prejudices have to be taken into account. To minimize the risk of unseemly and unscientific squabbles, no one can be immortalized on Mars until they are safely dead, preferably for a few

centuries. There could be no lobbying or infighting over the claims of such scientists as Copernicus, Darwin, Galileo, Sir William Herschel, Hipparchus, Huygens, Kepler, Mendel, Newton, Pasteur, Rutherford, Tycho Brahe . . . Great explorers like Columbus and Magellan were also honoured, and so was Leonardo da Vinci, presumably for his studies of flight – he appears to be the only artist on Mars.

Nearer to our own time are the Curies (Marie is the solitary woman – scandalous, because there have been many distinguished woman astronomers), Sir James Jeans (but not Sir Arthur Eddington!), Gerard Kuiper and of course Percival Lowell. It is amusing to note that his assistant Andrew Douglass, whom Lowell ultimately fired because of his scepticism about the 'canals', has a crater located a safe 400km distant from his ex-employer's. The Russian 'Chief Engineer' Sergei Korolev (whose name was never revealed to the West in his own lifetime) has, surprisingly, not yet been joined by Konstantin Tsiolkovsky; nor are Robert Goddard, Hermann Oberth and Wernher von Braun yet on Mars – though that will certainly be rectified in due course.

Three of the greatest science-fiction writers are already there: H. G. Wells, Jules Verne and their German counterpart Kurd Lasswitz, and so is Edgar Rice Burroughs. John W. Campbell seems at first glance to have been honoured as well; in fact, though, this is not the famous editor of *Astounding/Analog* magazine but a Canadian physicist of the same name. How ironic! In 1941 *this* John W. Campbell, then President of the Royal Astronomical Society of Canada, published a paper on 'The Problem of Space Travel' in the prestigious *Philosophical Magazine* (January 1941) 'proving' that a lunar spaceship would need an initial mass of 1,000,000,000,000 tons to make the round trip – grim news for the future of space travel indeed . . . had he not misplaced a few decimal points. Certainly the *other* John W. Campbell deserves to be on Mars, and I have made a strong plea to the IAU for his star author, Robert A. Heinlein, to be honoured as well.

I was pleased to discover that I knew personally two of the scientists now on Mars. One was the UK biologist and polymath J. B. S. Haldane, who wrote about space travel as early as 1927. In his essay 'The Last Judgement' (the final item in the still highly readable volume *Possible Worlds* [1927]) he rather conservatively put the first Mars landing in AD9,723,841. A couple of decades after the essay appeared, addressing the British Interplanetary Society on the biological problems of

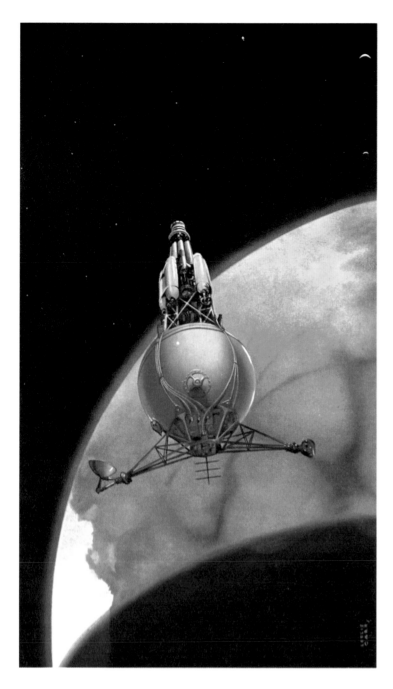

A robot Mars probe designed by R. A. Smith and painted by Leslie Carr; this painting was the frontispiece of my book *The Exploration of Space* (1951). Note that the probe contains all the basic features (camera, propulsion system, long-range antenna) incorporated into the *Mariner* and *Viking* probes a quarter of a century later.

spaceflight, he was prepared to move the decimal point several places. The other 'Martian' I knew was the brilliant aeronautical engineer Theodore von Karman, whom I met at conferences arranged by the International Astronautical Federation. As he was a co-founder of the Jet Propulsion Laboratory, to which we owe most of our real knowledge of Mars, it is altogether appropriate that he has a memorial on the planet.

The name on Mars for which I have the most affinity, however, is that of an obscure Englishman who died eight years before I was born. Major Percy B. Molesworth was an amateur astronomer who established an observatory on a highland overlooking the magnificent natural harbour of Trincomalee, on the east coast of Ceylon (now Sri Lanka). Through his 13in (33cm) reflecting telescope he made fine drawings of the Moon, Jupiter and especially Mars which were published during the early years of the century by the British Astronomical Association. He died on Christmas Day, 1908, at the early age of forty-two. A few years ago I located the remains of his little observatory. Staring eastwards across the Indian Ocean, as Molesworth must so often have done when Mars was rising, I wondered what he would have thought had he known that before the end of the century there would be a 175km crater bearing his name on the world to which he devoted so much of his short life.

Although they will be much further away from home, the first Mars explorers will have a considerable advantage over their precursors on the Moon; they will be able to 'live off the land' much sooner.

By the time humans reach Mars, robot orbiters and landers will have already given them a good idea of local resources. If water has been discovered, probably in the form of permafrost, the difficulty of establishing a Mars base will be enormously reduced. An alternative source of supply would be the atmosphere, but extracting the trace amounts of water vapour would require considerable amounts of energy and equipment.

Just as on Earth, energy is really the key to survival on Mars. The complete absence of free oxygen in the anyway very thin Martian atmosphere means that, even if life still exists somewhere on the planet (albeit not at the *Viking* landing sites), we cannot expect to find the equivalent of animals. Plants, algae, etc. – no problem. But the internal-combustion engines of fast-moving creatures like ourselves need oxygen to burn the fats and sugars that power them. Of course, one can imagine alternative biological machines, and the recent discovery of lifeforms based on sulphur reactions around Earth's deep ocean vents should remind us of nature's ingenuity. Nevertheless, in the very unlikely event that there are mobile Martians, they would probably make our tortoises and sloths look like race-horses.

The most readily available natural source of energy on Mars is solar, and it could be even more useful there than on Earth. Although the intensity of sunlight is less than half that on our planet, there are few clouds and, except during the huge dust-storms that occasionally veil much of the planet, very little atmospheric absorption to weaken it. So sunlight will be readily available for the generation of electricity and, even more important, for the growing of plants to provide food and oxygen. The combination of a carbon-dioxide-rich atmosphere plus water plus sunlight is a powerful one: it created the environment in which we now live. It may do the same on Mars, though hopefully over a timescale a few thousand times shorter.

As soon as possible after the landing, the first explorers should establish a 'garden on Mars', even if only a very small one. Conceivably this could be attempted by the earlier robotic missions, although it is difficult to imagine a robot having the necessary green thumb. The first Mars gardens would be inside small, inflatable transparent domes, held up by an internal pressure high enough to permit workers to use simple breathing gear instead of the full-body spacesuits required in the normal Martian environment. There is virtually no limit to the size of these domes; they could eventually grow large enough to enclose towns or cities.

The much publicized 'Biosphere II' experiment in Arizona, in progress as I write these words, had as one of its objectives the collection of information needed to establish a self-sufficient Mars base – or, for that matter, lunar base. The key phrase, of course, is 'self-sufficient': few human settlements would have survived very long on *this* planet if they had been compelled to import not only all their food but also every breath of air.

Although the architecture already looks a little dated, there is nothing intrinsically wrong with the Mars base I described in *The Exploration of Space* (1952) and also used as a background in the novel *The Sands of Mars* (1951):

Inside these great bubbles of air the colonists could live

exactly as they would on Earth: only when they ventured outside would they have to put on their breathing equipment. If desired, the domes might be made of some transparent, flexible plastic to let through the sunlight, though this is by no means essential and might result in too great a heat loss during the day. The best arrangement would be a dome which was transparent during the day, and so collected heat on the 'greenhouse' principle, and which could be made opaque at night.

. . . On the excellent principle of not putting all one's eggs in the same basket, there would be several small pressure domes rather than a single big one. They would be linked together with airlocks and there would also be locks in each dome communicating with the surrounding country-side.

. . . Although the 'weather' inside the domes would be completely under control, it would appear advisable to roof the buildings so that they could be individually pressurized. Thus in case of failure of the dome all the inhabitants indoors would be safe, and could go to the help of anyone who had been caught out in the open . . . The further domes [shown in the illustration] cover the chemical plant – where oxygen and other essential materials are obtained from ores and minerals brought in from outside – and the food-producing plant with its farm and processing equipment.

In the distance is the combined air- and spaceport. Here the atmospheric-type rockets land after making contact with orbiting spaceships . . . A jet aircraft is seen departing on a journey to another settlement: for short-range transport, pressurized vehicles with large balloon tyres would probably be used, as on the Moon.

Within such cities, the lives of the Martian colonists need not be unduly restricted or monotonous. Boredom would, in any case, be the least of their worries. Around them would be a whole world awaiting discovery – a world which will probably keep geologists, botanists and zoologists busy for centuries.

Over forty years later, that last sentence is still valid. Even if the 'botanists and zoologists' discover no trace of Martian biology, past or present, they will be fully occupied studying – and modifying – the terrestrial lifeforms transplanted to the New World.

4

Virtual Explorations

In 1955 I published a novel on which I had been working for more than twenty years: *The City and the Stars* (original version, *Against the Fall of Night*). It involved what at that time seemed very wild extrapolations of computers and artificial intelligence – which I put more than a *billion* years in the future! At the time I had seen only a couple of very primitive computers, each occupying a large room; today scientists and engineers routinely hold more powerful versions in the palms of their hands. My Eternal City, Diaspar, was maintained and preserved by supercomputers:

He waved toward the perfect, infinitely detailed simulacrum of Diaspar that lay below them.

'That is no model; it does not really exist. It is merely the projected image of the pattern held in the memory banks, and therefore it is absolutely identical with the city itself.' . . .

For the next hour Alvin sat before one of the vision screens, learning to use the controls. He could select at will any point in the city, and examine it with any degree of magnification. Streets and towers and walls and moving ways flashed across the screen as he changed the co-ordinates; it was as though he was an all-seeing, disembodied spirit that could move effortlessly over the whole of Diaspar, unhindered by any physical obstructions. Yet it was not, in reality, Diaspar that he was examining. He was moving through the memory cells, looking at the dream image of the city . . .

Yet it could show him something that no living man had ever seen. Alvin advanced his viewpoint through the grille, out into the nothingness beyond the city. He turned the control which altered the direction of vision, so that he looked backward along the way that he had come. And there behind him lay Diaspar – seen from the outside.

To the computers, the memory circuits, and all the multitudinous mechanisms that created the image at which Alvin was looking, it was merely a simple problem of perspective. They 'knew' the form of the city; therefore they could show it as it would appear from the outside.

It is not often that I can pinpoint the origin of my crazier brainstorms, but in this case I know exactly what gave me the idea for my hero's vicarious exploration. In 1948, during my final year at King's College, London, the Science Faculty's physics lecturer, Dr Mackay, gave a demonstration of what would now be called computer graphics. By today's standards it would seem childishly crude. The (monochrome, of course) cathode-ray tube displayed simple 'wire-frame' outlines of cubes and other basic geometrical objects. However, what made Dr Mackay's lecture so impressive was his ability to rotate these images in their electronic space and to look at them from any angle. None of our BSc Physics Finals class had ever seen anything like it. Here was something new – but who could have guessed at what it would lead to, in another thirty years?

The use of computers to simulate artificial or virtual realities is now an extremely active field of research, and today's video games only hint at the possibilities of the not-too-distant future. Although current artificial-reality systems are extremely expensive and quite crude, they enable one to have the sensation of walking through buildings which do not yet exist, and to explore places which never *could* exist.

The Artificial Worlds currently available are – at least to would-be explorers who do not have access to Pentagon funds – greatly limited by the size of computer memories and rates of processing information. To store a *single* full-colour image requires about a megabyte – the capacity of a high-density $3\frac{1}{2}$in diskette: the same diskette can easily hold the text of a long book. *One second* of animation, at the PAL standard of twenty-five frames a second, would require twenty-five diskettes! At the time of writing, not many domestic computers have hard disks capable of storing as much as half a minute.

Fortunately, the situation is not quite as desperate as this naïve analysis indicates. Clever 'image-compression' techniques have been developed which can increase capacity tenfold – even a hundredfold. Some of these depend on the fact that between the successive frames of a movie, or animation, only a small portion of the picture usually changes. So why regenerate a completely static background twenty or thirty times a second?

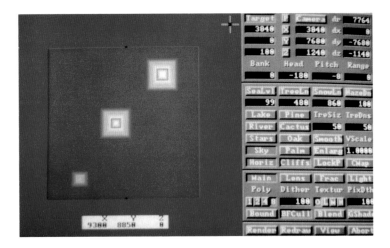

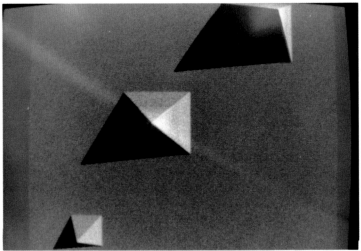

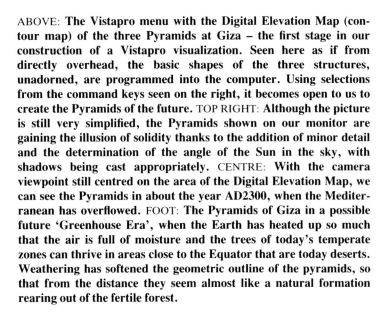

ABOVE: **The Vistapro menu with the Digital Elevation Map (contour map) of the three Pyramids at Giza – the first stage in our construction of a Vistapro visualization. Seen here as if from directly overhead, the basic shapes of the three structures, unadorned, are programmed into the computer. Using selections from the command keys seen on the right, it becomes open to us to create the Pyramids of the future.** TOP RIGHT: **Although the picture is still very simplified, the Pyramids shown on our monitor are gaining the illusion of solidity thanks to the addition of minor detail and the determination of the angle of the Sun in the sky, with shadows being cast appropriately.** CENTRE: **With the camera viewpoint still centred on the area of the Digital Elevation Map, we can see the Pyramids in about the year AD2300, when the Mediterranean has overflowed.** FOOT: **The Pyramids of Giza in a possible future 'Greenhouse Era', when the Earth has heated up so much that the air is full of moisture and the trees of today's temperate zones can thrive in areas close to the Equator that are today deserts. Weathering has softened the geometric outline of the pyramids, so that from the distance they seem almost like a natural formation rearing out of the fertile forest.**

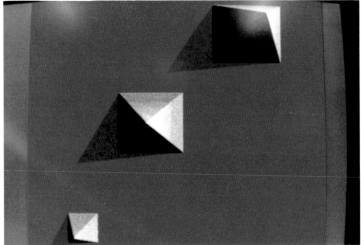

Even so, until recently the average home computer could show images of little more than cartoon-quality; photographic realism seemed utterly beyond reach.

No longer. Welcome to Vistapro.

In early 1990 Virtual Reality Laboratories of Ganador Court, San Luis Obispo, California, sent me a program for the Commodore Amiga called Vista 1.0. It was several months before I ran Vista, and a little longer before I realized that life

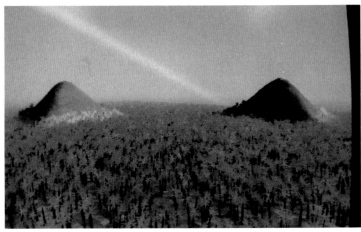

would never be the same again. Like Alvin, I had discovered something more interesting than mere reality.

The Vista program was developed by Hypercube Engineering's John Hinkley and Brick Eksten. What it does may be stated very simply: it enables one to create totally realistic images of a landscape using as raw material nothing more than a contour map of the terrain, encoded in digital form. The computer is instructed to behave like a camera, creating the view that would actually be seen, looking towards any point, from any position.

Suppose that Vista's subject were one of the oldest and most impressive of all human monuments: the Great Pyramid of Giza. It is difficult to think of any structure whose shape can be more concisely described: four identical triangles outlining a square 230m on a side, meeting at an apex 150m above the ground. If drawn as a contour map with height intervals of ten metres, it would look like fifteen squares nesting inside each other – a pattern that could be defined mathematically in binary code as a very few lines of 0s and 1s. With this 'description' loaded in its memory a computer could generate images of the Great Pyramid from any conceivable viewpoint. Given a location immediately above the vertex it would draw a square, given one at the centre of a face it would draw a triangle, and so on for intermediate positions. The mathematical operations involved are trivial – the solution of a few equations which even the cheapest of PCs could handle in seconds.

Such an image, however, would give no impression of solidity: it would be only a line-drawing – a so-called 'wire-frame'. A more sophisticated program would be needed to make the Great Pyramid appear a real, three-dimensional object. To do this the computer has to generate surfaces clothing the naked framework. The next step is to consider the lighting: you need to 'tell' the computer the position of the Sun. After a few more milliseconds of cogitation it decides that one face is brightly illuminated while the others are in shadow. Now the Pyramid does indeed look like a real, solid object – but it might just as well be a 10cm plastic model on the nursery floor. There is no clue to its scale, partly because it has no *texture*. Nor is there any way in which this could be displayed, given the fact that the computer has been loaded with nothing more than the Pyramid's overall dimensions, and has no information about its fine detail – such as the layers of carved stone blocks of which it is actually comprised.

For serious archaeological studies, this information has to be fed into the computer, perhaps by drawing the contour lines only a few centimetres apart. Obviously, this would require an enormous increase in the amount of data loaded into memory. The file on the Great Pyramid would now be kilobytes or even megabytes in size; no problem, but it would take correspondingly longer to generate new images. Maybe several whole seconds . . . However, there is a simple alternative if all you want to do is make beautiful pictures. There are computer recipes (subroutines) for generating any imaginable pattern or texture. It is a straightforward matter to call up the 'Blocks, large, assorted' program and clothe the Great Pyramid with a surface that would fool anyone except a professional egyptologist.

And, of course, there is no need to stop there; what you can do is limited only by your imagination. If you would like to see the Pyramid plated with gold or covered with a few acres of mink, that can easily be arranged. And what about that rather unusual tourist attraction – snow on the summit? Just set the 'Snow Line' in the computer at the 100m level and the result will be a miniature Everest-on-the Nile. Perhaps you would like to show the Pyramids in the Late Greenhouse Era, with only their tips peeking above the ocean? No problem: 'sea-level' can be set at any desired value, and everything below that will automatically be obliterated. You can even add waves to make the result more convincing.

Though the Vista program does not feature the Great Pyramid,* its latest version displays a considerably larger *natural* formation of roughly the same shape. This is the 230m-high Devil's Tower made famous by Steven Spielberg in *Close Encounters of the Third Kind* (1977). Because the Devil's Tower is a much more irregular object than the Great Pyramid the file containing the description of its basic geometry is fairly large, over 700k – big enough to hold a full-length novel of 100,000 words. I would defy even the Editors of *Reader's Digest* to describe every crevice and cranny of the Devil's Tower so well in 100,000 words that a *completely accurate visual image* could be recreated from them. Nor does the Vista program attempt this. It generates the outline of the hill to a precision of a few metres and then fills in the details from its imagination.

*I sent these paragraphs to John Hinkley for his approval, and he took my thought experiment seriously. He looked up the dimensions of *all* the Giza pyramids and encoded them into Vistapro. With the disk he sent I was able to turn my *imagined* virtual reality into – well – *real* virtual reality, with the results shown on page 46.

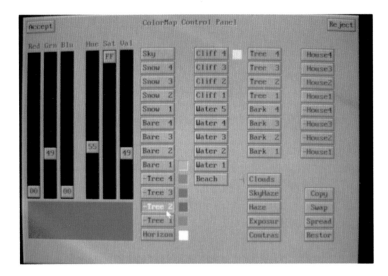

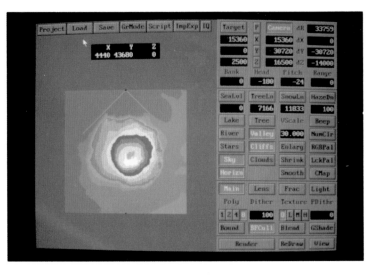

The basic tool-kit by use of which the Vistapro renderings reproduced in this book were created: an expanded section of the menu, showing some of the settings – horizon, cloud-cover, sea-level, treeline, snowline and many more – which control the image rendered by the computer. (*Courtesy John Hinkley*)

Alongside the Vistapro menu, the Digital Elevation Map of the central caldera of Olympus Mons; all the near-view renderings of the great volcano reproduced in this book were based on this map. The area shown is 150 kilometres square.

To explain how it does this would require an extended detour into the realms of Chaos and fractal geometry. However, there is an example of the technique involved which everyone must have used at one time or another, especially in infant school. When children draw a house or a landscape, they often fill up the otherwise blank spaces by scribbling over them. If done properly, the more scribbles, the more real the scene appears to become. By the use of simple programs, the computer can be told to 'scribble' in ways that, though completely random, give very convincing results. Most people viewing the image of the Devil's Tower created by Vistapro 2.0 would believe that they were looking at a genuine colour photograph. But the fine details of the surface are completely imaginary, existing only in the memory of the computer. Any rock-climber who used the image to plan a route to the top would be in real trouble after only a few metres.

The original Vista program provided, on a single diskette, the information from which images of several famous terrestrial landscapes could be generated; they included Crater Lake, Yosemite and, perhaps the most striking of all, Mount St Helens both before and after its devastating 1988 eruption. Most of the beauty spots in the United States are now available on disk; the basic information comes from the Geological Survey's DEM (Digital Elevation Model) files which map the continent at intervals of thirty metres.

However, though it is interesting to survey the breached summit of Mount St Helens and to flood (or drain) Crater Lake, I very soon turned my attention to more exotic terrain – Mars. The Vista files contained the data not only for the largest volcano in the Solar System, Olympus Mons, but also for the 4000km-long canyon Mariner Valley (Valles Marineris) which runs parallel to the equator for a quarter of the planet's circumference.

The Vista 1.0 databank for Olympus Mons contained only the central caldera, a 'mere' eighty kilometres across; as we saw (page 27), it closely resembles Kilauea except that it is about ten times larger and could swallow the entire island of Hawaii. It formed an ideal target for my initial exploration of Mars – and my sometimes laborious ascent of the Vista program's learning curve (Vista is user-friendly, but not foolproof). Though few things are more frustrating than reading software manuals without being able to play with the hardware, I will try to convey the excitement of my first raids on Olympus Mons:

When the MONS.DEM image is called up it is not much to

look at – merely a contour map tinted in the usual convention, with the lowest areas shaded dark and the highest ones light. By clicking the mouse on CAMERA a point of view can be selected anywhere in the map's 6000 square kilometres, and from any altitude – even from so far out in space that Olympus Mons is no more than a pimple on the face of Mars. The mouse is then clicked on TARGET, which determines the point the camera is aiming at. Now the program can be started by selecting RENDER, and after a few seconds the image will flash on the screen.

In that short time, the computer has solved literally millions of problems in solid geometry, working out the shape of the landscape as it appears from the selected viewpoint. It has also done a similar number of calculations to decide, from the position of the Sun in the sky, the distribution of light and shade. To do this in a reasonable time for every one of the more than a million pixels (picture elements) displayed on the monitor would be impossible except for a supercomputer, so the Vista program divides the scene into myriad small triangles or polygons, and assigns some fixed value to each one. The result is an electronic mosaic: the image appears to be built up from thousands of little tiles, no two adjacent ones the same.

This crude 'quick look', which is generated in a few seconds,* allows you to decide whether this is the picture you really want. Usually it is not, because viewpoint and camera angle will seldom be right at the first attempt. In fact, they are often hopelessly wrong, because of what my friend HAL was fond of calling 'human error'. Examples include putting the camera underground, or aiming it straight up at the sky. However, such accidents are often very serendipitous: they frequently produce delightfully bizarre effects that would never have been discovered by a really expert operator.

Once the first rough sketch of a landscape has been rendered by the computer, you are faced with an immense variety of choices or options, for various programs allow you to manipulate the image in an almost infinite number of ways. All the

*My Amiga 3000 with Progressive Peripheral's 68040 accelerator board takes about fifteen seconds to produce the lowest-definition 'quick look'. High-resolution images, especially with added features, may take up to an hour. Fortunately the computer can be set to do overnight runs, storing ten to twenty images for viewing at breakfast-time. Most of the renderings reproduced in this book were in fact done using the MS.DOS version of Vistapro on a Compaq Prolina 4/50.

possibilities of even the relatively simple Vista 1.0 program could not be exhausted in a lifetime; there must be quadrillions of combinations of target-and-camera positions alone.

Like a tourist visiting a foreign country for the first time, I wandered around the Olympus caldera taking snaps in all directions, and saving the best ones to send home. I also made a few raids into Valles Marineris, but its sheer size and complexity challenged my ability to find any dramatic compositions. With Olympus Mons, it was difficult *not* to.

One day, while I was inside the crater looking up at the towering walls around me, I had a brilliant idea. If I moved the point-of-view of the 'camera' a few hundred metres and got the computer to generate a second image, I could make a stereo pair and produce a 3-D effect! I tried it, made a series of colour transparencies of the VDU screen for various separations, and spread them out on a lightbox. Then I examined sets of right-and-left images with a little stereo viewer – appropriately enough, the one tucked in the back cover of NASA's *Viking Orbiter Views of Mars* (1980). To my delight, it worked perfectly – especially for landscapes under a star-studded sky. When I deliberately transposed right and left images, the stars appeared to be *closer* than the distant horizon! So my stereo technique was really working . . .

My elation was cut short when I came across an article in the September 1991 *Amiga World* by science and science-fiction artist Joel Hagen, 'Fantastic Voyages: Creating a Mars Simulation'. He had been using Vistapro for months – and had also been generating stereo images . . .

After a few weeks of playing with Vista I had become so addicted that, when I learned that it had been superseded by the greatly improved Vistapro, I simply had to get hold of the new version. Here are some of the Vistapro options available when the camera position and point-of-view have been selected, before the command is given to generate ('render') a landscape:

○ You can supply a sky of any colour, and sprinkle it with stars.
○ You can create rivers and lakes; the water-level will be set automatically to the contour line selected. Then you can make the water any colour you like. Finally, waves and ripples can be added.
○ Snow can be placed on high ground, above any designated contour line.

○ Selected areas can be tinted to indicate trees or vegetation. A palette mixing green, red and blue provides an almost infinite range of colours.

○ Trees ('fractal' – but convincing – oaks, pines, palms and cacti) can be planted in specified areas. Tree density and height can be set to any value.

○ Atmospheric haze, from faint to impenetrable, can be generated, giving a realistic impression of distance.

○ Surface texture can be modified from smooth to rough by subprograms invoking fractal mathematics.

○ The apparent focal length of the camera can be varied from wide to zoom, giving an enormous range of magnifications.

○ The vertical scale can be adjusted to flatten or exaggerate the terrain being viewed.

These are only the main options provided by this amazing program; after months of playing with it I am still discovering others.* Once an image has been generated, it can be discarded if it does not live up to expectation, or saved to be played back at leisure. A high-resolution picture may take over a megabyte of storage space, so serious explorers will require the biggest hard disk they can afford.

More than two years after I had been slowly climbing up the Vistapro learning curve, John Hinkley sent me his latest

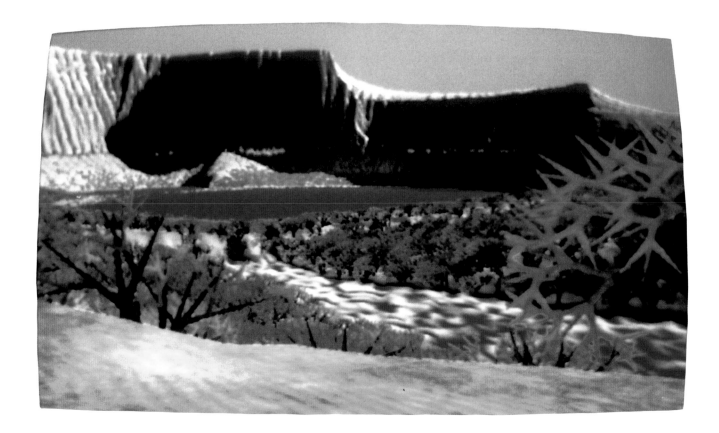

The caldera of Olympus Mons in about the year AD4000, according to a Vistapro projection by the author. Blue skies, tranquil lakes and verdant slopes deceive today's eye into seeing this as a view of Earth; only the lack of erosion along the ancient yet sharp cliff-edges betrays the scene as being certainly set upon another planet.

*I should emphasize that no knowledge of computer theory, still less of mathematics, is needed to operate Vistapro. The basic principles can be mastered in a few hours, and my assistants were soon producing such dazzling pictures that I had to practise hard to keep up with them.

production – Mars Explorer – on a single CD/ROM disk. As soon as I had installed it, I was hooked. Never in my wildest dreams had I imagined that one day I would sit at a computer keyboard and wander at will over the ravaged face of Mars, looking down upon its craters and ravines through the robot eyes of the *Viking* space-probe . . .

The program is incredibly easy to use: it opens with the rust-red globe of the planet, looking almost three-dimensional, slowly revolving against the blackness of space. Though only a few details, such as the great chain of Tharsis volcanoes, can be identified, it is sobering to realize that no astronomer ever had such a clear view of Mars through any telescope on Earth.

For close-ups of the planet, it is necessary only to set the cursor on the selected area of the map shown in the main menu. And if you wish to find a feature whose location you do not know, clicking the mouse on the list of names will bring it up automatically on the screen.

You can then 'fly' over the face of Mars, using the scroll arrows, and increase the magnification from ×4 to ×32. The highest power will show objects about a kilometre across – it would take weeks to examine every detail that is shown. (Nevertheless, I cannot help dreaming of the treasure that was lost with *Mars Observer*, which might have improved our maps a hundredfold.)

It soon became a challenge to see how well I could match the *real* Martian landscapes with those generated by Vistapro. The palette allows one hundred distinct settings of forty-five independent parameters, and I leave it as an exercise to the student to work out the number of possibilities: I doubt if the lifetime of the Universe would be sufficient to explore them all.

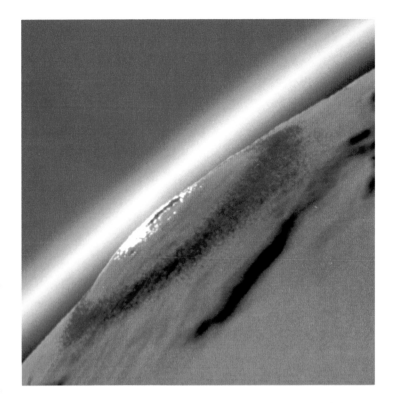

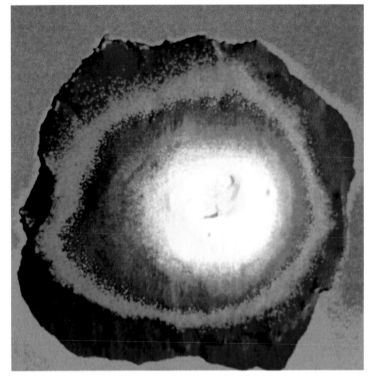

TOP: **Dawn over Olympus Mons in the year AD3500 is as spectacular as any scene on Earth could be – and all, at least on the planetary surface, to a far greater scale. Note how, even at this distance, bands of vegetation in the foothills of the mountain give texture to the otherwise largely featureless plains.**

FOOT: **A further rendering depicting a far-future Mars, perhaps two millennia after the commencement of terraforming. Now the mighty Olympus Mons has become merely an island amid the great (but shallow) Olympus Sea. The vegetation colours – with the white of the montane icecap in the centre – give us a living key to the mountain's contours.**

Much of my Amiga's hard disk is now devoted to Olympus Mons, seen from all angles – not only as it is now but as it was a few billion years ago and, much more important, as it may be a few centuries in the future, when the long Martian winter is brought to an end.

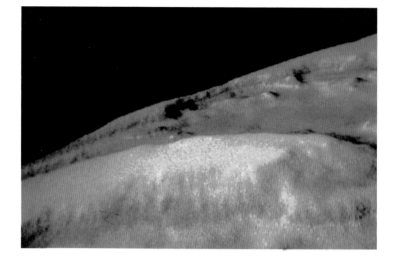

Ophir Canyon as it might appear today (RIGHT) and the same scene after seven centuries of a determined terraforming program (BELOW). What the bright colours of the vegetation – lichens in the higher regions, trees, bushes and grasses in the lower ones – disguise is the fact that it is still bitterly cold for almost all of the year.

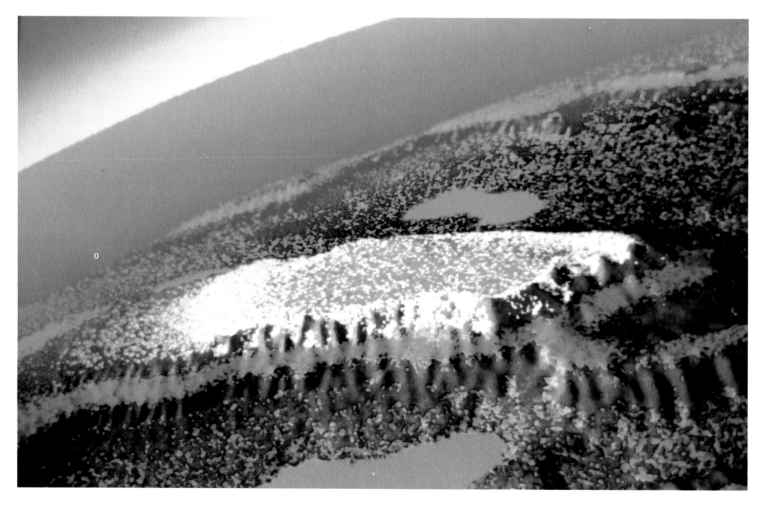

PART II

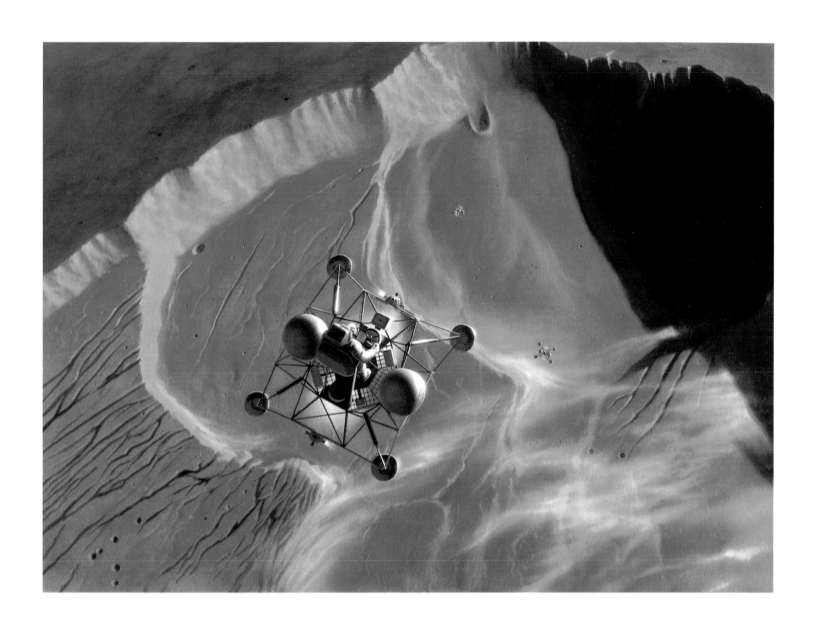

ADVICE TO MARS TOURISTS

For artistic reasons, the vertical scale of most images in this videochip has been exaggerated by a factor of three. To avoid disappointment, anyone planning a safari (real or virtual) should therefore consult the local guides for the best (and safest!) scenic routes. Armchair explorers should also remember that insurance on robot telesensors can be very expensive.

Welcome to Mars! – Public Relations Department,
Port Lowell, Democratic Republic of Mars
(third edition, 2061)

PREVIOUS PAGE: *Fieldwork*, **by Pat Rawlings. In the early days of the exploration of Mars, a flight of single-pilot hoppers descends into the great caldera of Olympus Mons.** (*Painting by Pat Rawlings, reproduced by permission*)

5

The Snows of Olympus

Olympus Mons is the tallest mountain in the Solar System . . . Its average slope angles only five degrees above the horizontal, but the circumference of the lava shield is a nearly continuous escarpment, a roughly circular cliff that drops 6km to the surrounding forests. The tallest and steepest sections of this encircling escarpment stand near South Buttress, a massive prominence which juts out and divides the south and south-east curves of the cliff. There, under the east flank of South Buttress, one can stand in the rocky upper edge of the Tharsis forest, and look up at a cliff that is twenty-two thousand feet tall.

Kim Stanley Robinson, *Green Mars* (1988)

Well, yes – but there's a problem here, and we'd better face it before we go any further. Although Olympus Mons is awesome, it is not, except in a few regions, *spectacular*. A comparison of its profile with that of Everest shows why: some ninety per cent of its surface area is a gently sloping plain. You could be almost anywhere and never guess that you were indeed standing on the 'tallest mountain in the Solar System'.

The only really dramatic features of Olympus Mons are the central caldera and the surrounding escarpment, so I naturally concentrated on those for my portrait gallery. And even here I must confess that I, ahem, cheated a little.

The 'Digital Landscapes' stored in the Vistapro files have a threefold vertical exaggeration, so that all slopes look much steeper than they actually are. It is easy to correct this by using the program's 'scaling option' to divide by the same factor, and thus flatten out the landscape to show it as it would really appear. Alas, all too often the result is quite dull and uninteresting.

What to do? After much soul-searching, I decided that, after all, I am not a Martian real-estate salesman who might be answerable to the local Chamber of Commerce. ('Spectacular view of the sheer Tithonis cliff-face from your picture window!') It also seems to me that the expression '*virtual* reality' gives me a good excuse for imaginative artwork; so I freely admit that in the Martian portrait gallery on the ensuing pages I have put aesthetics before science. My qualms of conscience have been further assuaged by the fact that JPL has gone to much worse extremes. Its spectacular Mars and Venus 'Movies', generated by programs essentially the same as Vistapro, employ even larger vertical exaggerations – so much so that one critic has said: 'They'd make the average house look like the Washington Monument.'

This may be a good place to mention an error sometimes made by artists depicting lunar or Martian scenes. It is natural to assume that, in a lower gravity, the angle of slope of broken rock (talus), sand or other granular material would be much steeper than on Earth. Not so; because the horizontal frictional force which prevents sliding depends *directly* on the downward thrust due to weight, the value of gravity cancels out. Surprisingly, therefore, the angle of slip for any given material would be the same on an asteroid – with, say, one-thousandth Earth gravity – as on a neutron star – where the surface gravity would be measured in tens of *billions* of gees!

But enough of this quibbling: now let us admire one of the grandest formations in the Solar System.

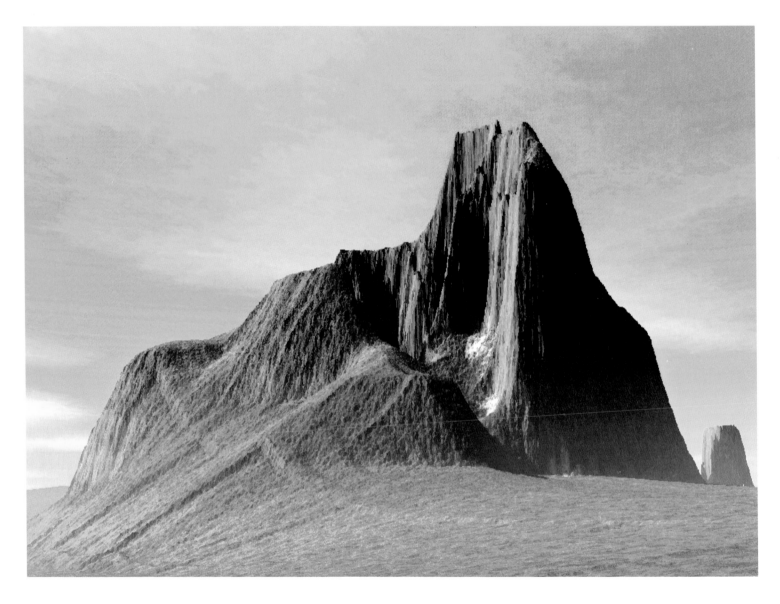

Southeast of Olympus Mons, the Tharsis region contains the three other great volcanoes of Mars – Ascraeus Mons, Arsia Mons and Pavonis Mons – as well as countless smaller ones. This Vistapro rendering by John Hinkley shows one of the lesser peaks of the Tharsis area beneath the salmon Martian sky. (*Rendering courtesy John Hinkley*)

ABOVE RIGHT: **A sight no human being has yet seen, but given to us through the workings of Vistapro: dawn over the foothills of Olympus Mons.** (*Rendering courtesy John Hinkley*)

OPPOSITE: **Profiles of Mount Everest and Olympus Mons, drawn to the same scale. Although the great Martian volcano is some three times higher than Earth's tallest mountain, it is obvious that height alone is the least important factor in comparing the two.**

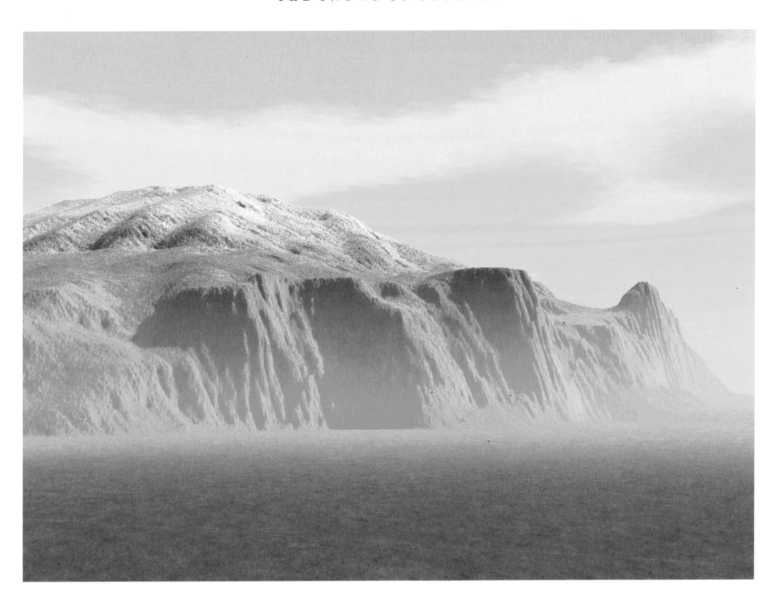

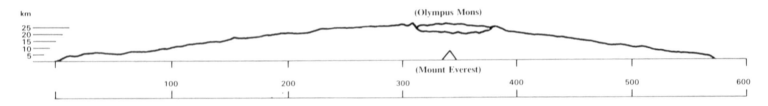

The year is AD3000. Because of its elevation, Olympus Mons was the last region of Mars to become terraformed; indeed, many colonists – the 'Reds' – vigorously resisted the idea and tried to preserve the volcano in its original state. Of course, they failed . . .

In this view, which covers an area of almost a million square kilometres, a hardy green lichen is beginning to spread upwards from lower ground, and there is a sprinkling of H_2O (water) snow around the central caldera, twenty-five kilometres above the surrounding plain. However, the 'Olympian lakes' (see page 72) still lie centuries in the future.

Compare this Vistapro-generated image with that on page 27, which shows Olympus Mons as it is today. Both have a vertical exaggeration of about three times.

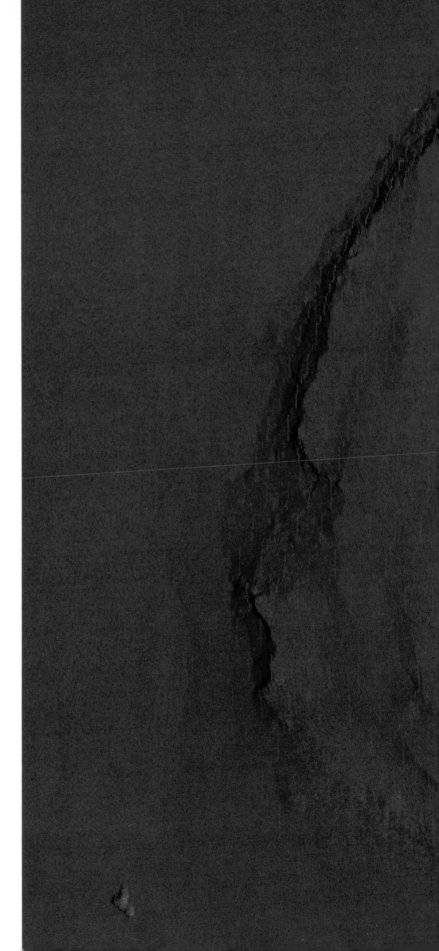

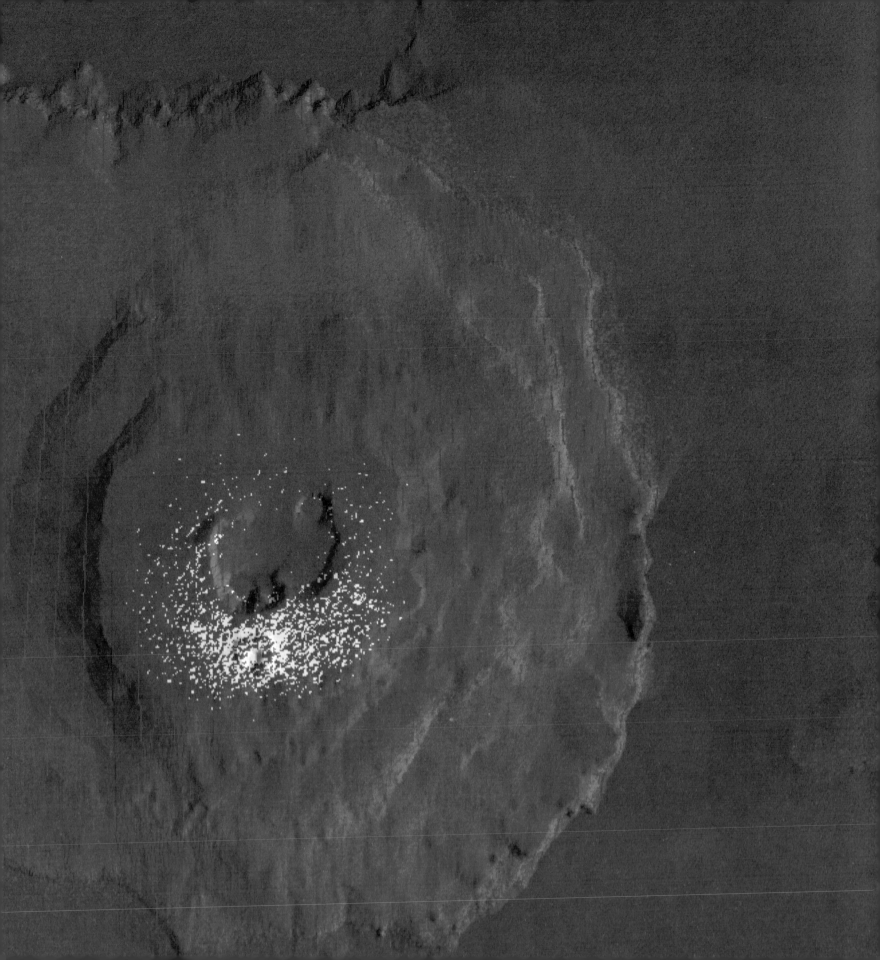

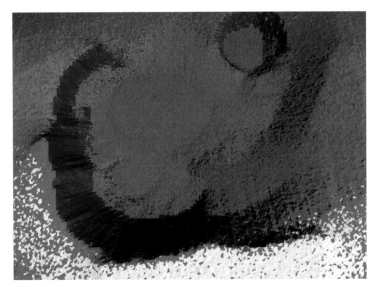

LEFT: **The *Viking*'s-eye view of Olympus Mons' central caldera, at an elevation of almost twenty-five kilometres above the surrounding plain. The area shown is more than one hundred kilometres wide: it is large enough that it could enclose Earth's entire island of Hawaii – with *all* of its huge volcanoes.**

During the nineteenth century Earth-based astronomers, with remarkable prescience, gave this region the name Nix Olympica ('The Snows of Olympus') as it often appeared a brilliant white. What they observed was actually its extensive cloud cover; but there probably is snow here from time to time – though of carbon dioxide rather than H$_2$O (water).

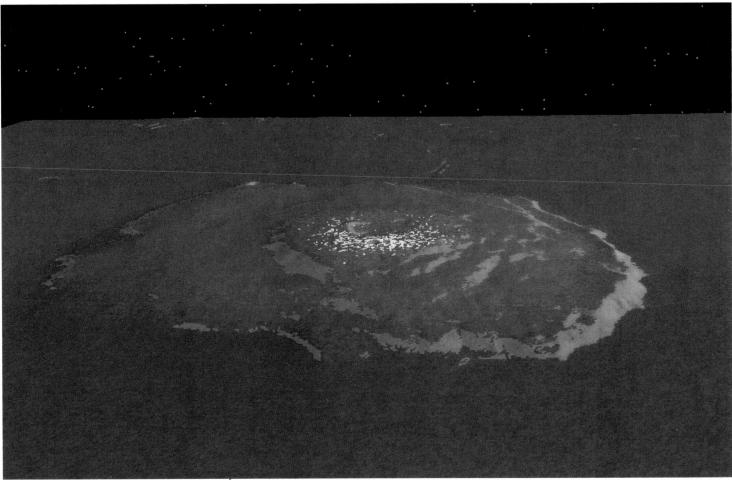

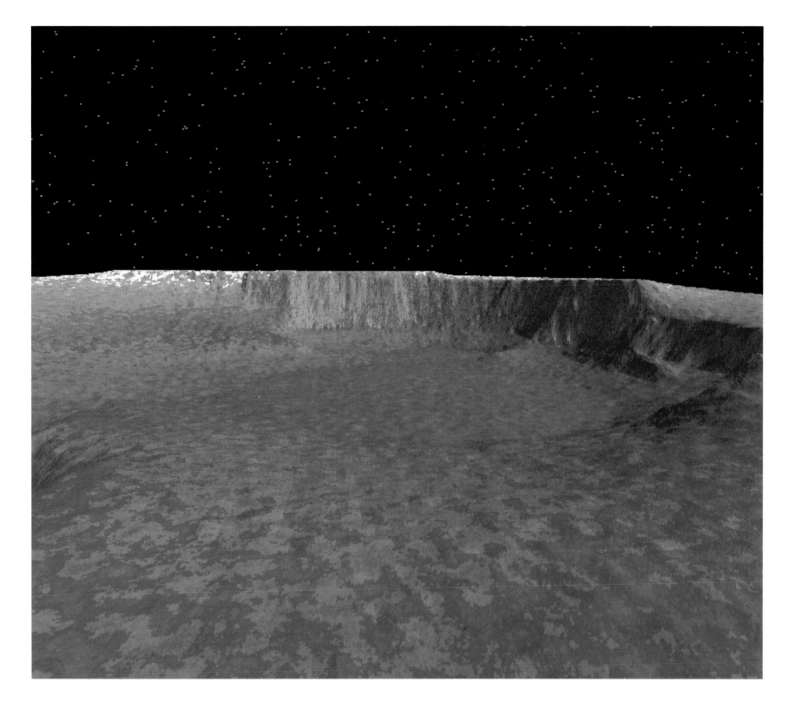

OPPOSITE: **Mons Olympus as it might have been observed from the** *Viking* **orbiter when it was heading towards the north. There is considerable vertical exaggeration in this image – see page 69 for an image rendered to show a more realistic profile of the surrounding cliffs.**

ABOVE: **The view across the central caldera of Olympus Mons as it is today. Owing to the absence of atmospheric haze at this altitude it is virtually impossible to judge distances visually, but the far wall of the crater is more than fifty kilometres away.**

ABOVE: **Approaching Mons Olympus from the south in about AD2100, soon after terraforming has started and the first lichens have begun to spread over the surrounding plain.**

OPPOSITE TOP: **One hundred or so years on from the previous scene, terraforming lichens have invaded the caldera and the atmosphere is becoming thick – as evidenced by its increasing blueness. The Earth's sky is blue during the day but red at sunrise** and sunset due to the differential scattering of the light from the Sun by dust and other particles suspended in the air; the blue of the Sun's light is more easily scattered than its red, which is why we see predominantly red when we are looking through a greater distance of atmosphere at the rising or setting Sun. Before terraforming began the Martian atmosphere was loaded with huge quantities of dust (sufficient, during the height of the wild dust-storms, to blot out the sky), and was consequently a salmon-pink colour.

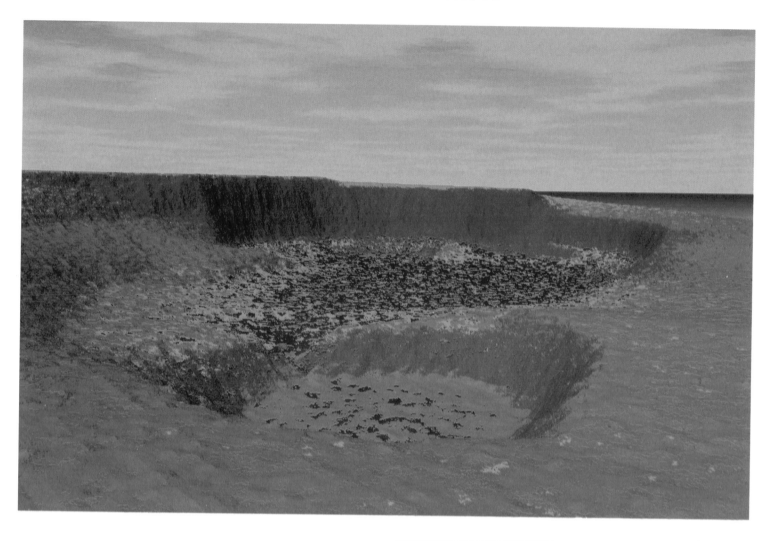

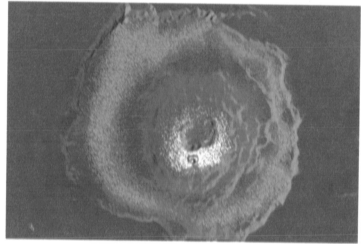

RIGHT: **AD2200, and the greenbelting of the mountains has begun, with different varieties of lichens and primitive plants finding the altitudes that best suit them. For most of the year, however, the temperature is far below the freezing-point of water, and on the highest ground even some carbon-dioxide snow still persists.**

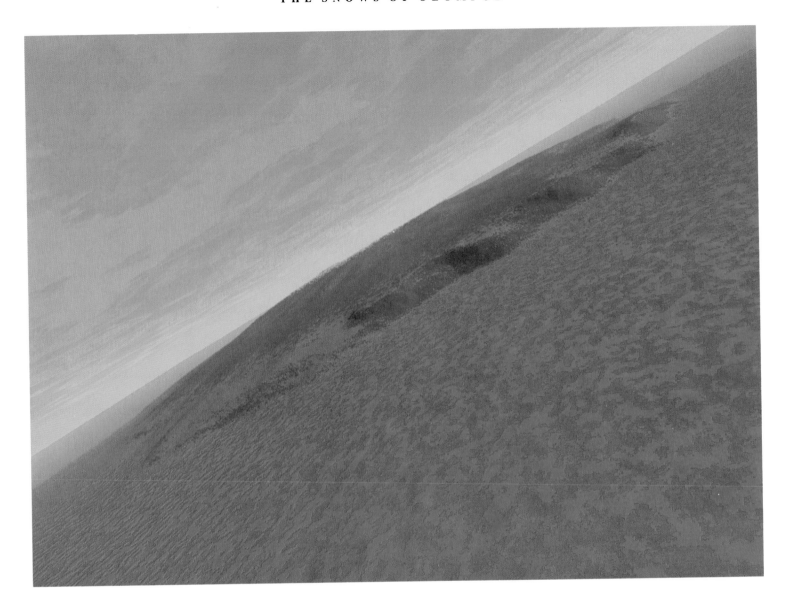

ABOVE: **The same view as shown in the image on page 62, but about one hundred years later. Much of the plain surrounding Olympus Mons is now covered with a wide variety of different plant lifeforms. Although the atmosphere has become considerably denser over the intervening century, it is still unbreathable by imported terrestrial animal lifeforms, except for a few specially developed – and very slow-moving – insects and others.**

OPPOSITE TOP: **The foothills of Mons Olympus in the year AD2300. This view of Olympus from the south has been rescaled in the** computer to show the true gradient of the approach – unlike the case in some of the earlier images, where gradients were exaggerated in the interests of clarity and, to be honest, dramatic effect.

OPPOSITE: **A view in the same general region and era as the preceding image, but in greater close-up. Contrary to some reports, the ascent to the Mons Olympus caldera does not present a serious challenge to mountaineers . . . indeed, members of the local bicycle clubs are fond of demonstrating that there are very few routes up the mountain which they aren't prepared to tackle.**

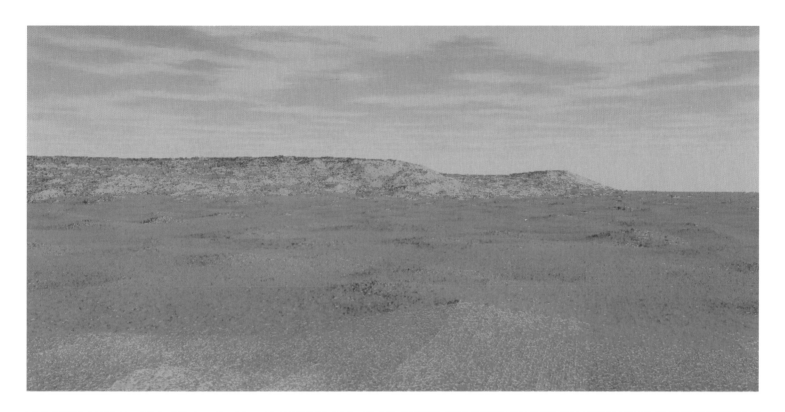

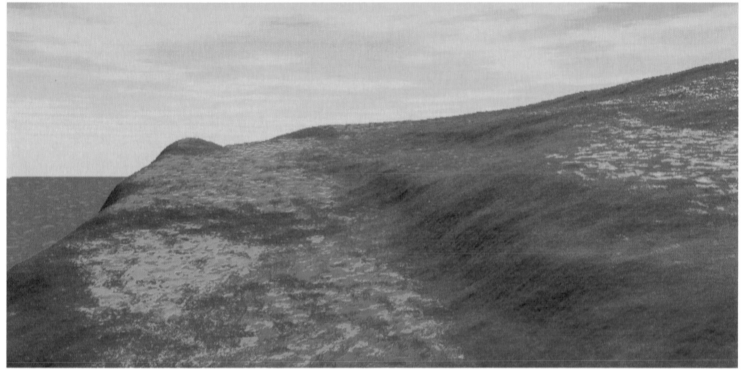

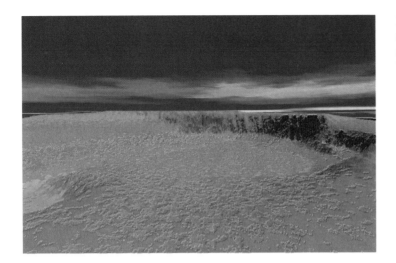

LEFT: **It is now AD2400, and red and green lichens are slowly spreading over the floor of the caldera – which, like most volcanic soil on Mars as on Earth, is rich with the chemicals necessary for the promotion of life.**

BELOW: **About one hundred years later than the previous scene, the floor of the caldera is no longer entirely dominated by lowly plantforms such as lichens. Now we can see a sprinkling of the first generation of Mars-growing pines – precursors (although pines will eventually, centuries hence, lose in a contest with oak trees) of the woods that will soon surround the lake or lakes formed in the caldera.**

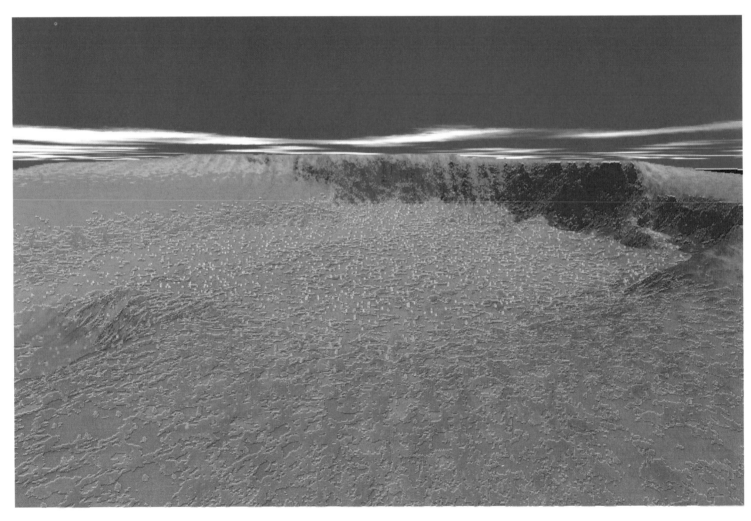

RIGHT: **In AD2500, adopting one particular future scenario, there is a single large lake in the caldera of Mons Olympus – and, because temperatures at this altitude are still very low as a result of the atmosphere's thinness, the Martian Winter Olympics can be held at any time of the year, even in the height of summer. A few redoubtable athletes have skated the full width of the lake, a stunt that will not remain possible, at least in summer, for more than a few decades longer.**

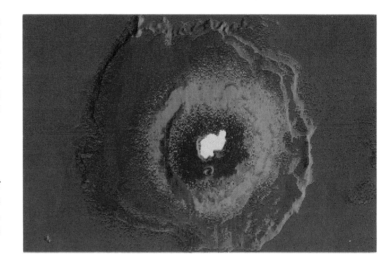

BELOW: **One hundred years later, in AD2600, during the height of the northern summer the temperature, even at this altitude, rises above the freezing-point of water, so that Lake Olympus thaws. Sailing here has become a popular sport – although icebergs are a major hazard.**

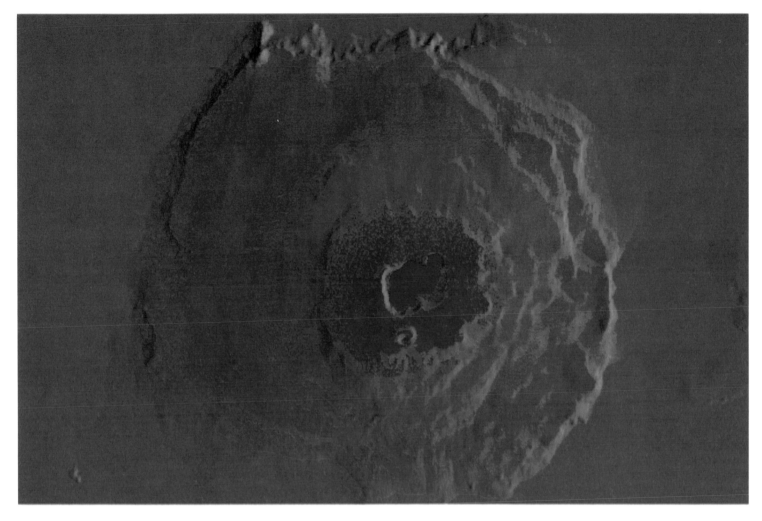

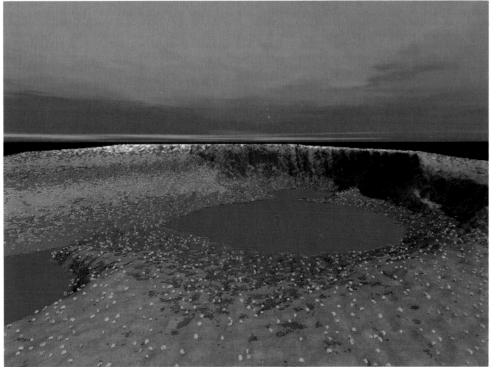

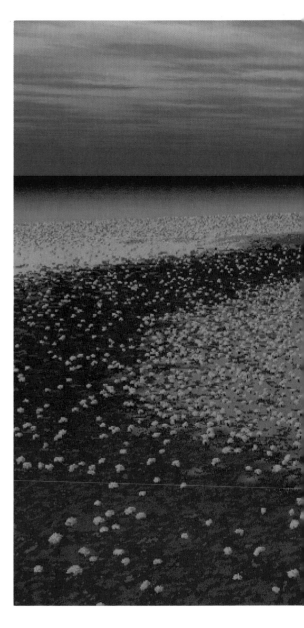

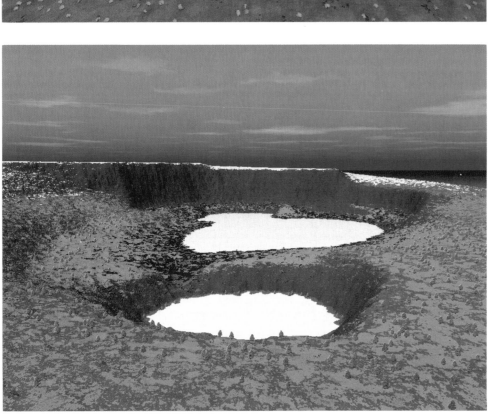

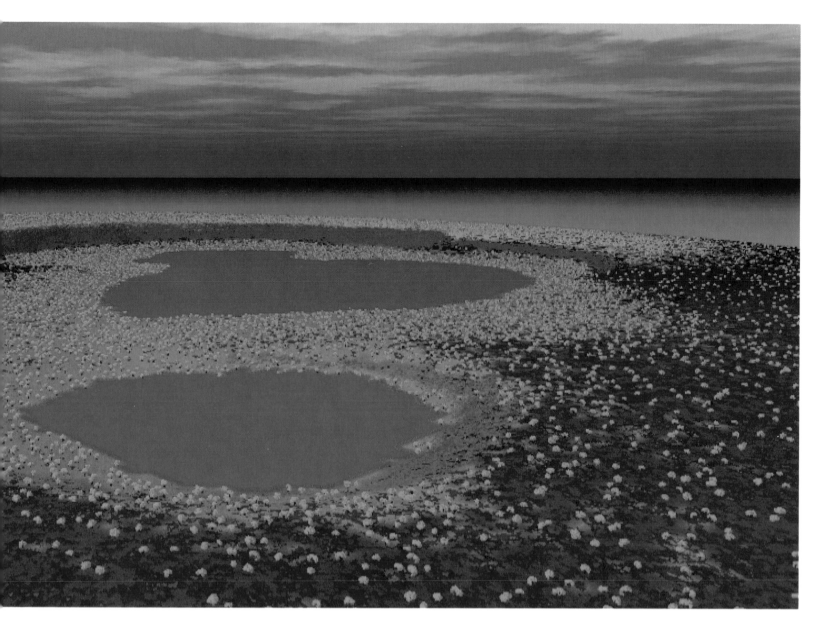

OPPOSITE TOP: **AD2700 and, with the rapid warming that is taking place all over Mars by now, oaks (i.e., deciduous trees) are beginning to replace the pines (i.e., conifers) on the floor of the Olympus Mons caldera.**

OPPOSITE: **Another possible scenario for AD2700. The fact that, for most of the year, the shallow Olympian lakes are usually frozen is a matter of great delight, of course, to those hardy colonists who enjoy winter sports. Even in the low gravity, however, skating is not particularly graceful when one is encumbered by a dozen kilos of**

life-support system – for at this altitude the atmosphere is still unbreathable . . . and for humans will probably never become otherwise.

ABOVE: **This image of the central caldera has been rescaled in the vertical direction (by comparison with the preceding picture) to show the surrounding walls more realistically. Even so, the scene is impressive: do not forget that the distance to the horizon is greater than fifty kilometres.**

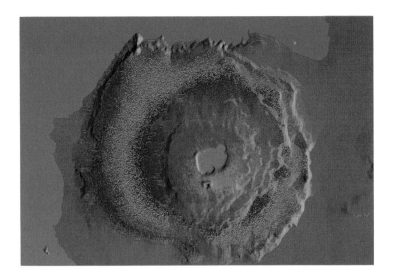

The spreading seas of Olympus. LEFT: AD2900: with the melting of the polar icecaps as a response to the advent of terraforming, large areas of Mars have now become flooded, and shallow seas are forming in many regions. BELOW: Summer in the year AD3000. The water has risen over the century that has passed since the last picture, and the shoreline has moved closer to Mons Olympus, which is now largely covered with flourishing vegetation. Sailing on these shallow seas has become, as it is on the mountain's caldera lake during summer (see page 67), a popular sport – but even at these lower altitudes it still presents dangers owing to the unstable weather conditions as the Martian climate continues to evolve. OPPOSITE: Half a year later, and the northern winter has the region in its grip. During the long winters the Olympus Sea – its waters almost pure, with only a negligible salt content – is completely frozen. At least another century must pass before year-round ambient temperatures will be high enough for fish to survive in these waters.

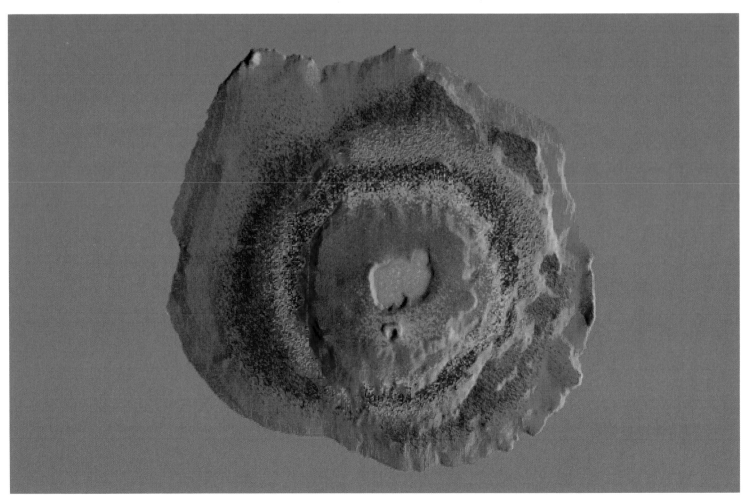

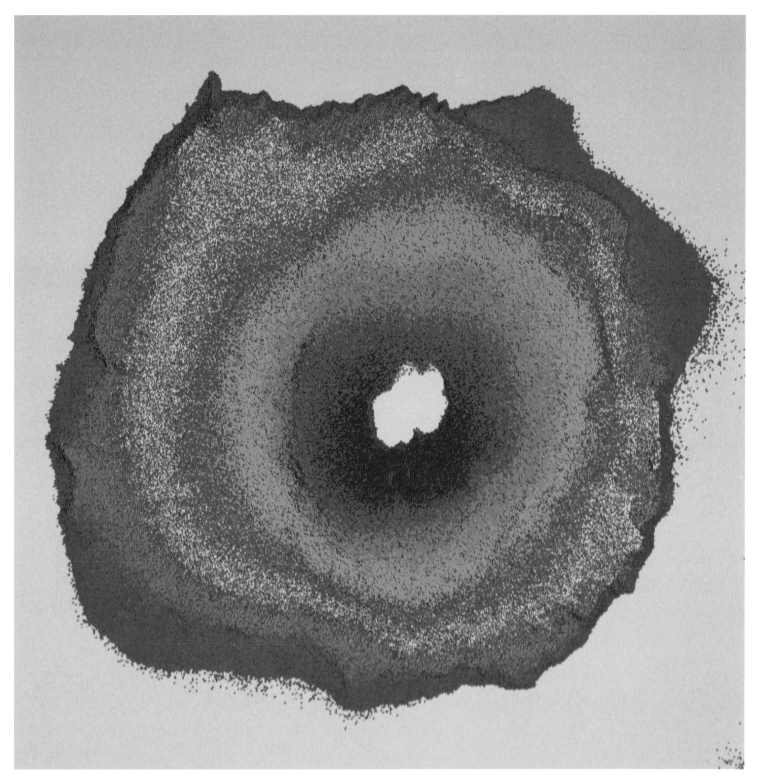

A sojourn much further into the future: the year is now AD4000. The atmosphere is dense enough for water to exist in the liquid phase all year round, even at this altitude, and the (very shallow) Olympian lakes are a permanent institution; they are supposed to offer the best fishing on Mars, and are much patronized by effete townsfolk, anxious to recapture something of the pioneering spirit of their ancestors.

Mutated oaks and pines – the latter stretching to more than one hundred metres in height – still co-exist, but the equilibrium between them is unstable: in a few more centuries the pines will be gone, unless for some reason the terraforming fails and goes into reverse . . . a possibility that causes a seemingly permanent heated debate over Marsnet.

(This image was created by John Hinkley, the inventor of Vistapro. The 'oaks' and 'pines' were fractally generated from a few lines of code, but the rendering itself took several hours, even on a fast PC. The slope of the caldera wall has been greatly exaggerated, and some of the apparent detail is in fact an artefact of the image-processing.) (*Rendering courtesy John Hinkley*)

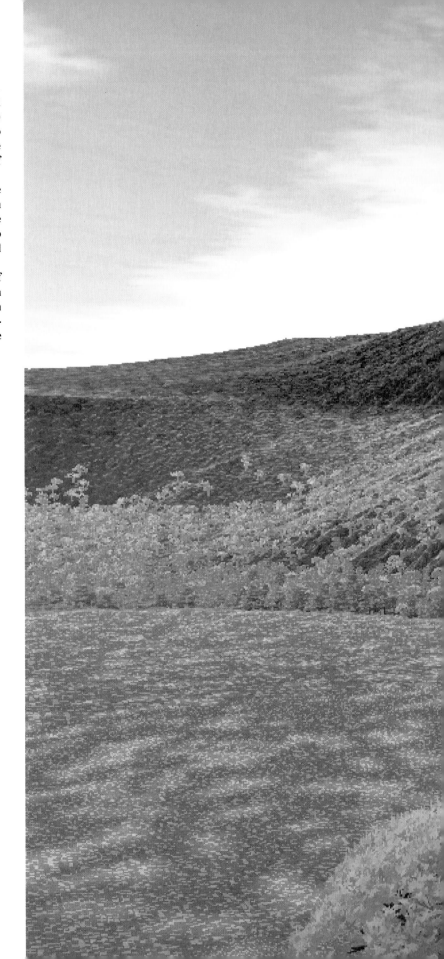

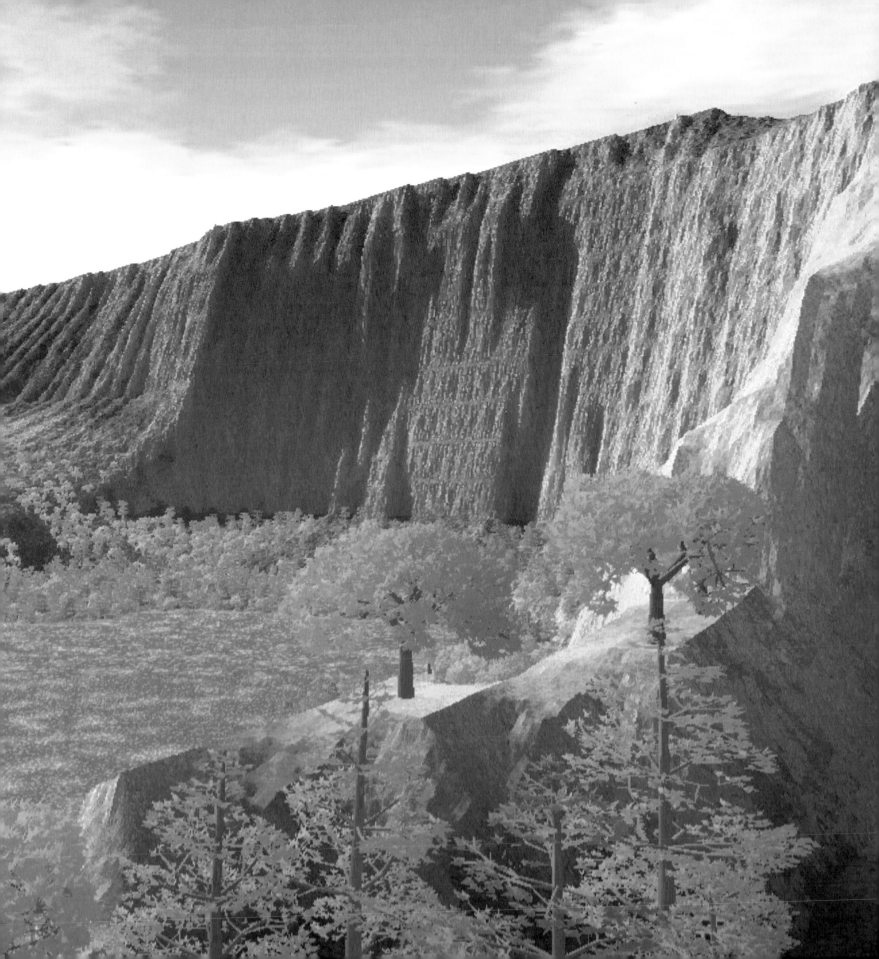

6

The Chasm of the Dawn

Valles Marineris is composed of steep-walled canyons, individually measuring up to 9km deep, 250km wide and 1000km long. They were named for *Mariner* 9, the Mars-orbiting spacecraft that took the first pictures of the canyon in 1971. The entire Valles Marineris system extends over 4000km from west to east near the Martian equator, and its size dwarfs all similar terrestrial features except, perhaps, the 5000km-long midocean rift system.

Viking Orbiter Views of Mars, NASA SP-441, 1980

The astronomers of the nineteenth century had a lot of fun naming the Martian features they dimly saw (or thought they saw) after classical gods and goddesses. Their Space Age successors have been happy to continue exercising their imaginations, though with much more justification. Thus the extreme eastern end of the enormous Valles Marineris complex has been christened Eos Chasma – the Chasm of the Dawn. A few hundred kilometres to the west are chasms with the equally romantic names of Ophir, Gangis and Capri.

Geologists – or, to be pedantic, areologists – are still not certain how this huge gash across the face of Mars was created. Although there are tributary canyons leading into the main valley, strongly suggestive of river-drainage patterns on Earth, water may not have played any part in their formation. It seems more probable that Valles Marineris is a gigantic fault, produced when the crust of Mars was torn apart by tectonic forces. (The Great Rift Valley of East Africa is a terrestrial example.)

Nevertheless, good arguments can be found to support the idea that water did in fact play some landscaping role in the remote past, when Mars perhaps had an atmosphere dense enough for it to exist in the liquid state. In particular, some parts of Valles Marineris show regular layering, typical of sedimentary processes. Once lakes may have existed in these now dry and dusty canyons; and, one day, they may return . . .

The entire length of the Valles Marineris is stored by Vistapro in 160 separate Digital Elevation Model (DEM) files, each of about sixty kilobytes, and representing an area 200km square. These squares form a rectangle extending for twenty units east–west along the equator and four units to its north and south. As this rectangle includes not only the Valles but the two giant volcanoes Pavonis Mons and Ascraeus Mons, it covers the most spectacular scenery on Mars. (Olympus Mons lies 600km further west, and is stored in another sixteen DEM files.)

Landscapes can be created from any one of the individual 200-kilometre-square digital maps, or adjacent regions can be joined together in 2 × 2 or 4 × 4 blocks to cover wider fields. In this way it is possible to select scientifically or aesthetically interesting domains of up to 800km on a side – just enough, for example, to cover the whole of Olympus Mons and not merely (!) the caldera on the summit.

Eos Chasma is actually a very broad valley, about 300km wide and 500km long, connecting two large areas of incredibly jumbled territory. Such Badlands, known as 'chaotic terrain', are common on Mars, and may have been formed by the widespread collapse of more ancient landscapes. Alternatively, they may be the product of catastrophic floods, for which there is a good evidence on our own planet. But the Martian floods, if they did indeed occur, must have been on a scale not seen on Earth since the end of the last ice age. Some calculations suggest that the peak flows must have been a hundred – even a thousand – times that of the River Amazon!

So where did all this water go? That is a very good question –

and one of the first that the next generation of robot probes will seek to answer. One plausible guess is that it is now bound up in Mars' polar caps or frozen in permafrost that perhaps lies not far below the surface of much of the planet – or, likely, both. In Chapter 8 we will discuss ways of mining it – and raising the temperature of Mars until the planet's water is liquid again.

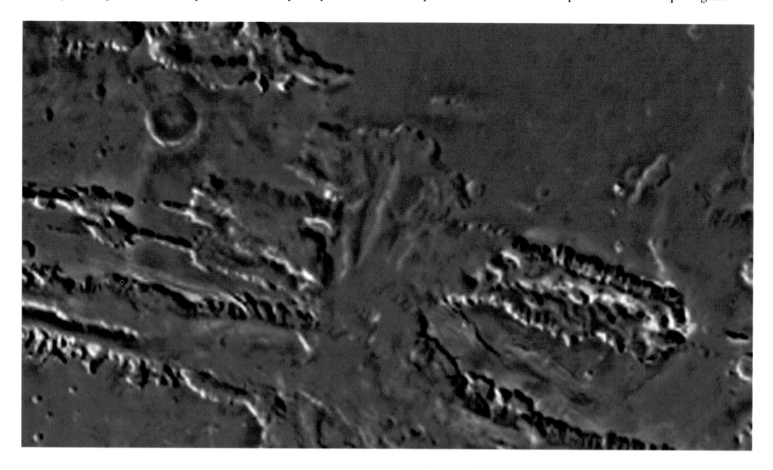

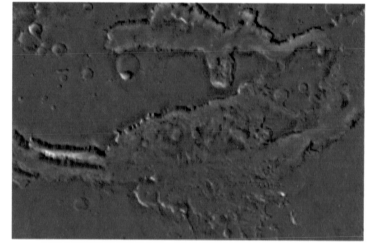

ABOVE: **This 1976** *Viking* **orbiter image shows an area of 1200 × 900 kilometres in the central region of Mariner Valley (Valles Marineris). Ophir is at the upper left: note how at some point in the past it has been breached by an enormous flood, presumably of water. Two hundred kilometres to the south, Coprates Chasma extends eastward into Eos, seen in more detail in the** *Viking* **image (RIGHT), showing an area of 1000 × 800 kilometres. This is at the eastern end of the Mariner Valley, where it opens out into Eos Chasma, the Chasm of the Dawn. Both of these images have been extracted from John Hinkley's** *Mars Explorer* **CD-ROM, which allows one to examine most of the Martian surface at varying resolutions down to a few kilometres. NASA's lost** *Mars Observer* **would have provided us with hundreds of times as much detail in selected areas. Hopefully, simpler and cheaper spaceprobes despatched within the next few years – perhaps based on demobilized 'Star Wars' technology – will be able to do this.**

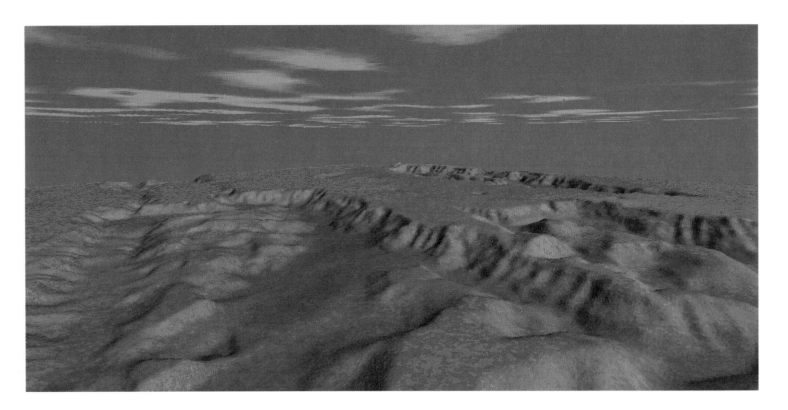

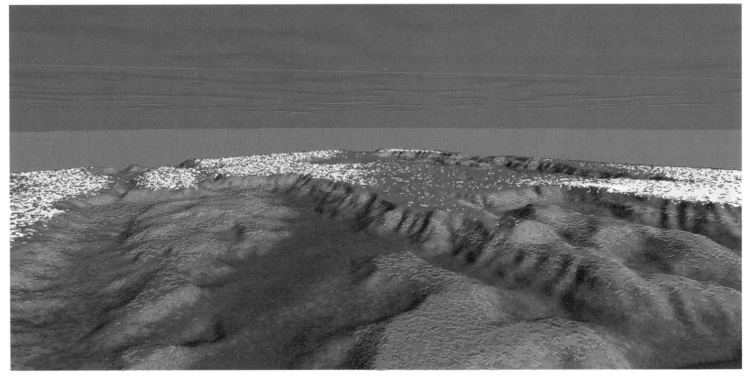

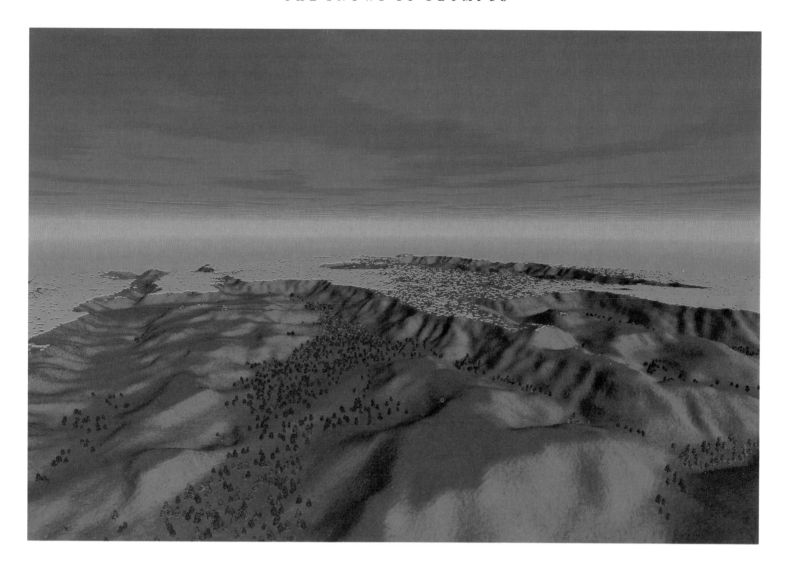

OPPOSITE TOP: **In the year AD2200 terraforming has just begun in Eos Chasma, at the eastern end of the Mariner Valley, and a few hardy lichens have begun to spread over the lowest areas. The dusty, salmon-hued sky is still much as the *Viking* lander saw it in 1976, but the degree of cloud cover, while still scant by terrestrial standards, is steadily increasing.**

OPPOSITE: **The same view as in the preceding image, but one hundred years later. The removal of much of the dust from the atmosphere has created a blue, almost Earth-type sky, and free water – although still only in the form of frost – is becoming more abundant. Various types of vegetation – green, pink and brown – are spreading over the landscape, releasing oxygen into the atmosphere. Although it is not yet possible for unprotected human beings to venture into the open, the wearing of full pressure suits is no longer necessary.**

ABOVE: **Another century has passed, and the year is now AD2400; we are looking out on the same view as in the two preceding pictures. A robust green grass covers much of the high ground, and giant Martian oaks, over one hundred metres tall, are conquering the valleys.**

Thanks to the extensive vegetation, the atmosphere's oxygen content has now reached ten per cent. This is still much too low for humans to be able to breathe the air, but a simple O_2 concentrator – not much bulkier than the first scuba gear *without* the tanks – allows the Martian humans virtually unlimited access to the open spaces of their world.

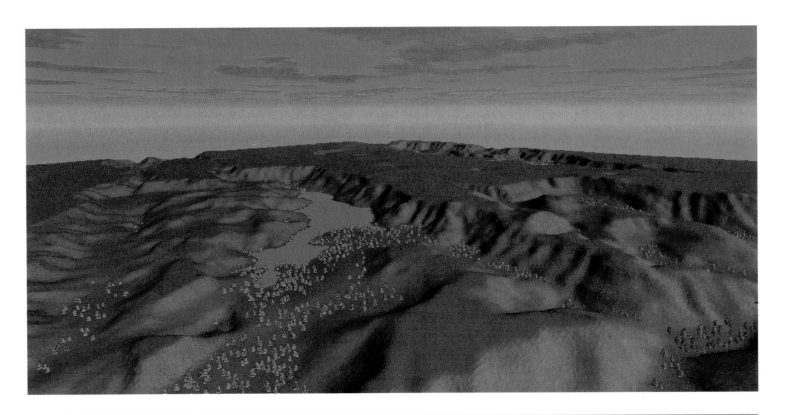

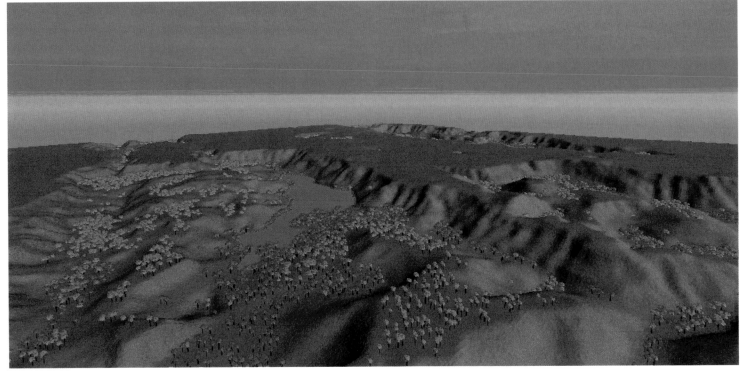

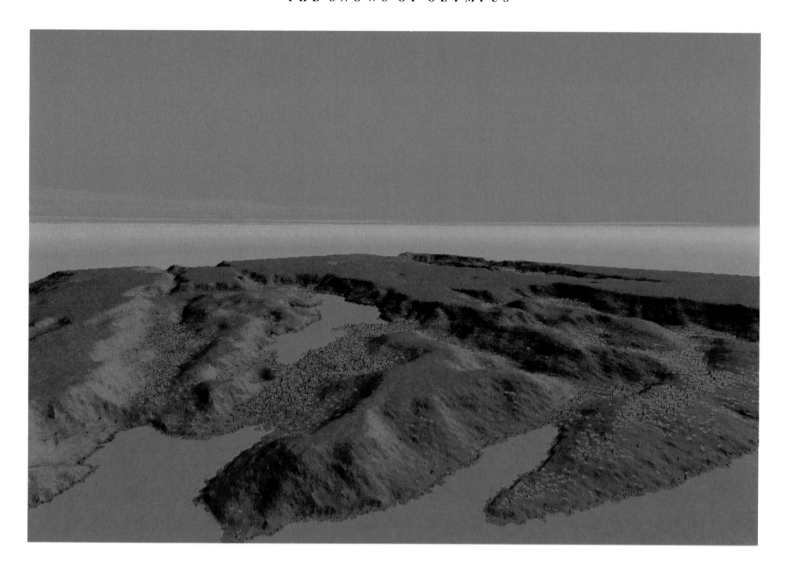

OPPOSITE TOP: **Three hundred years later, and the atmospheric pressure is now high enough for water to occur naturally in the liquid state, so lakes have begun to form in the lower valleys. Usually they are frozen, but at the height of summer – when the temperature may reach as high as ten degrees Celsius – there is a brief thaw. This is a time of great joy, for it heralds the era when there will be real oceans on Mars. Also in the lower valleys, a scattering of pines and oaks, co-existing but in an unstable equilibrium, surround the lakes.**

OPPOSITE: **The year is AD2800: a further century has passed since last we saw this scene. Now the Martian oaks are spreading out of the valleys and even conquering some of the higher ground; in this**

region at least, they have defeated the pines in the silent battle that has raged between the two tree-types over the past several centuries. The lakes now remain unfrozen throughout the summer, and attempts are being made to stock them with fish brought here in embryonic form – at great expense – from Earth's Antarctic regions.

ABOVE: Billions of years ago there were oceans on Mars, and now at last, in the year AD3000, those oceans are returning. The ocean currently flooding into Eos will eventually reduce it to a pattern of islands (see page 82, upper picture). The scale of the picture can be judged from the fact that some of these Martian trees are an astonishing quarter of a kilometre in height.

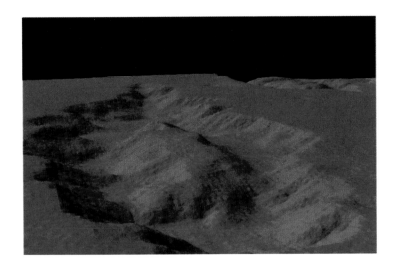

LEFT: **A typical view across one of the valleys branching out from Eos as it is today, a century or more before the beginning of terraforming. The region is utterly lifeless – more so than even the serest of Earth's deserts. But, by a few centuries later** (BELOW), **in the year AD2300, the scene has already changed considerably. Green lichens, capable of withstanding exceptional climatic extremes, are spreading over the landscape, while on higher ground H_2O (water) frost makes its appearance. However, the atmosphere is still very tenuous, so that water cannot yet occur in its liquid state. The first invasion of the area by trees still lies a hundred years in the future.** OPPOSITE TOP: **That century has passed, and the region's earliest trees are beginning to appear. The atmosphere, now denser, is changing from its original Martian salmon-pink to a more Earth-like blue – which many of the planet's human inhabitants find quite unpleasant. Two types of lichens – green on the high ground, red on the lower – are preparing the soil for higher forms of plant life.**

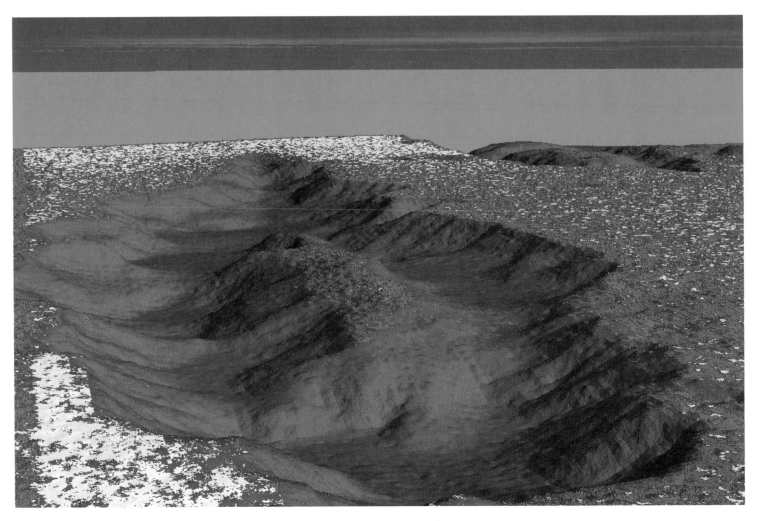

BELOW: **AD2500:** the centuries travel very swiftly when you are travelling through time by means of this limited form of Virtual Reality! Now the atmosphere is yet denser: the first lakes have formed and mutated pine trees are spreading, while the green and red lichens vie with each other on the higher ground. The red lichen – which people call the 'Red Weed' after the infestation in the novel *The War of the Worlds* by the long-ago Earth author H. G. Wells (a popular classic, alongside Ray Bradbury's *The Martian Chronicles*) – will eventually emerge the victor, at least until the pines invade its territory as oaks take over the lower areas from them.

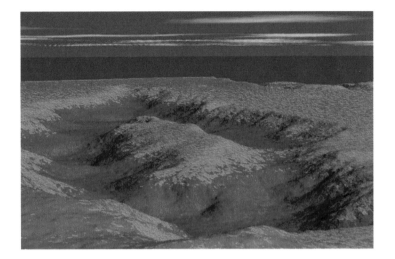

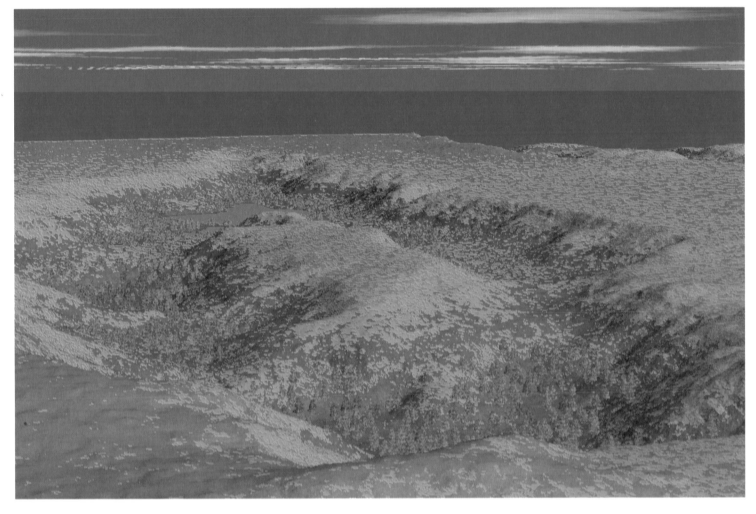

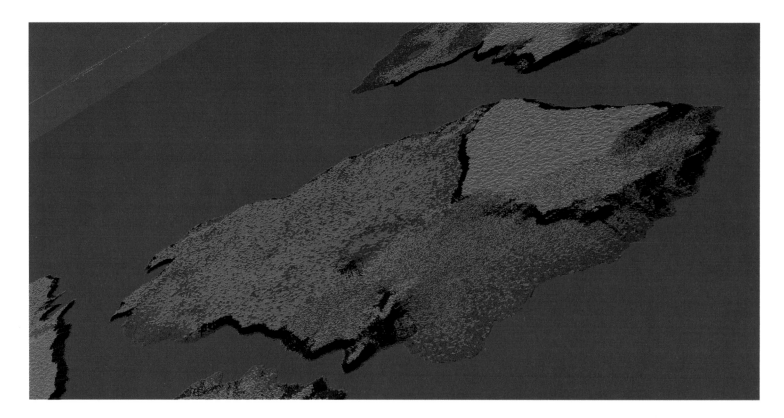

ABOVE: **With the centuries-long flooding of Mariner Valley, higher regions have been cut off to form islands – like this one at the end of Eos Chasma. These are the most fertile areas of the New Mars, and are covered with the nearest approximation this planet has to the Earth's tropical rainforest – although little of the vegetation growing here would be recognizable to an old-style terrestrial botanist.**

RIGHT: **AD4000. One of the New Martians' greatest pleasures is watching, through their network of survey satellites, the tide of life spreading across their world. They have never forgotten how their ancestors, more gloomily, used the same technology to monitor a somewhat similar process, but in reverse: the devastation of the home planet (although that term is little used today, since only visitors to Mars can think of any other world as being 'home'). This view of the long-flooded Eos Chasma from an altitude of one hundred kilometres is among most people's favourites, owing to the abundant and varied vegetation. Also visible are at least five fossil meteor craters, some of which now provide picturesque lakeside resorts.**

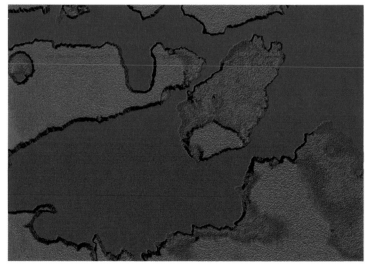

OPPOSITE: **A *Viking* image showing an area of approximately 900 × 600 kilometres of the western end of Mariner Valley – the westward extension of the areas shown in the pictures on page 75. This is the region named long ago by Earth-based astronomers as Noctis Labyrinthus – 'The Labyrinth of Night'.**

7

The Labyrinth of Night

It seems a pity that no Martian Minotaur can ever have roamed the Labyrinth of Night, which is large enough to swallow its namesake on Crete a million times over. A complex network of criss-crossing valleys, it covers an area about 500km long and 200km wide. At dawn, it is often filled with clouds; thin though it is, the atmosphere holds significant amounts of water, probably in the form of fine ice crystals which the heat of the morning Sun turns into vapour.

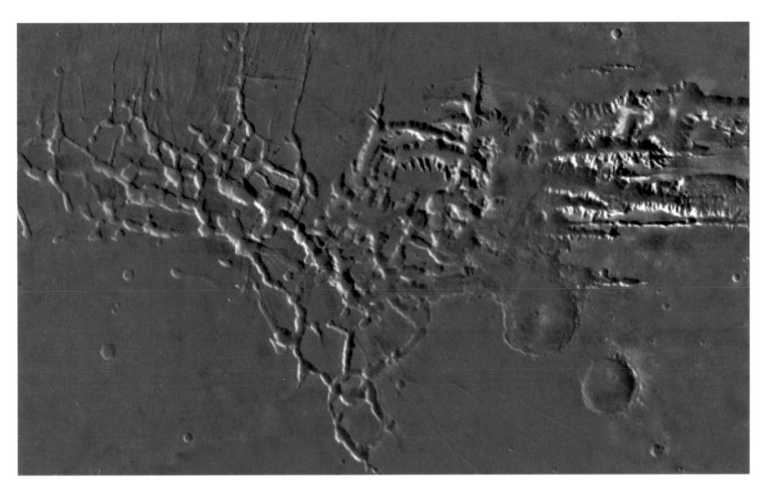

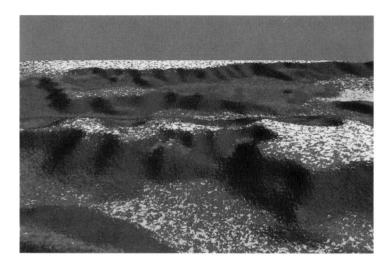

Looking across the western end of the Labyrinth of Night we can see that lichens are beginning to spread in the valleys now that – in AD2200 – the early stages of terraforming are well under way. There is H_2O (water) frost on the higher ground, although carbon-dioxide frost still persists there as well.

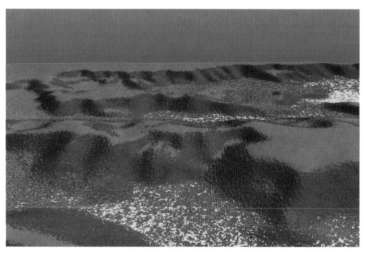

Two centuries later, in AD2400, the highlands are no longer covered with frost, and the sky is turning blue as the atmosphere becomes denser through the influence of terraforming.

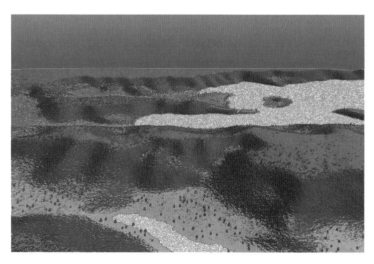

With the passage of another century of terraforming, higher plant forms have begun to appear in the area, with pine trees starting to grow in the valleys. Here and there lakes are forming, though as yet they remain frozen. It is a scene which occasionally makes recent immigrants from the wilder cold-temperate regions of Earth feel rather homesick – though Mars has yet to experience, and hopefully never *will* experience, the kind of heavy pollution that has devastated so much of even the remoter parts of their home world.

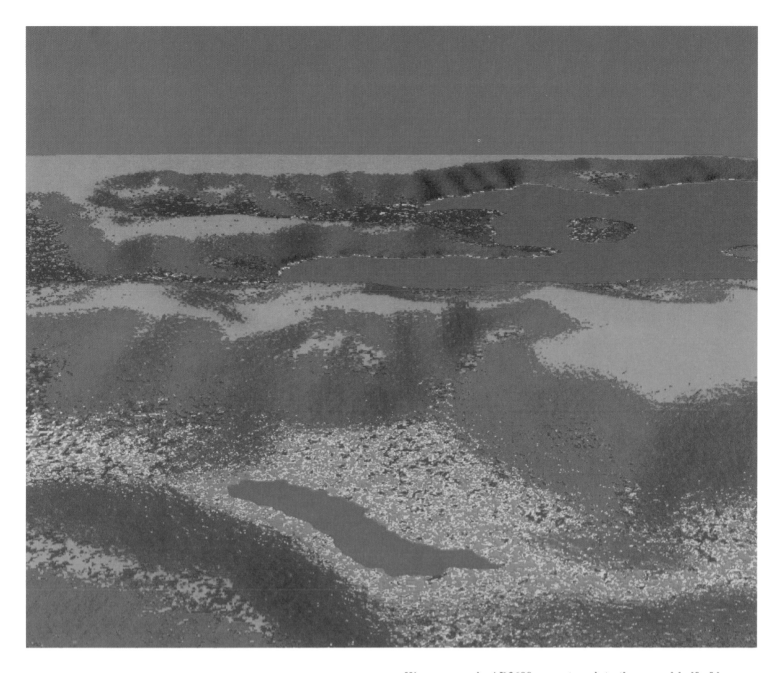

We are now, in AD2600, a century into the second half of human-kind's 'Third Millennium', and the terraforming of our species' second planet is continuing apace. Here in the Labyrinth of Night plant life of various kinds is spreading over the valleys, while the lakes scattered here and there across the landscape, though shallow, rarely freeze.

RIGHT: **Shifting our viewpoint away from that in the preceding set of pictures, here we see a different perspective across the Labyrinth of Night during the early days of terraforming, in AD2200. As elsewhere in the region, the first lichens and mosses are beginning to spread on lower ground. Back on Earth these plants would be regarded as the humblest of all, but here on Mars their annual progress is a matter of great satisfaction to the planet's human inhabitants – and a triumph for the scientists involved in the terraforming program.**

BELOW: **By AD2300 higher plants are taking over the territories once occupied by their more primitive precursors. The process may seem slow but, thanks to the help of the New Martians, the current rate of evolution here on the blossoming world is a full million times faster than ever it was on Earth.**

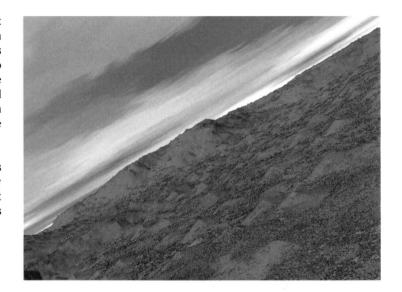

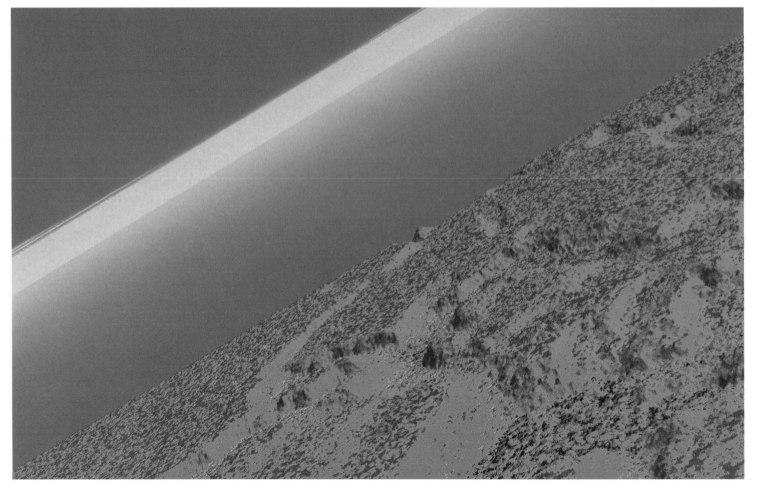

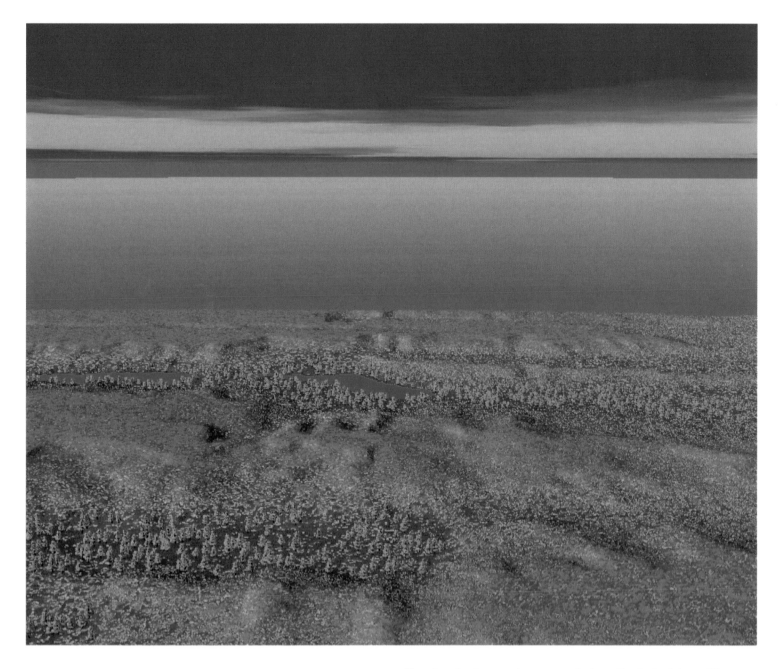

Two hundred years have passed since the last picture. Pines are almost ubiquitous in the more fertile areas of Mars, and the Labyrinth of Night is no exception: the trees, phenomenally tall by terrestrial standards, are forming clusters across the landscape, breaking up what was once a tract of dreary desert. As in other parts of the world at this latitude, small lakes are forming.

Looking down on the Labyrinth of Night as it is today from an altitude of one hundred kilometres. At dawn the valleys are often filled by mists forming from the H_2O (water) frost and carbon-dioxide frost on the higher ground. As the day progresses and the temperature climbs towards zero degrees Celsius – occasionally even past it – these mists disperse.

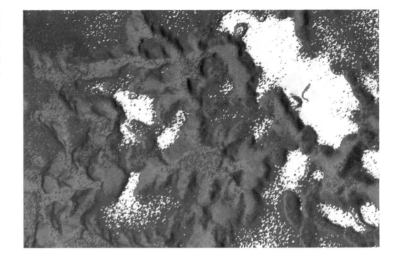

AD2300. After a few centuries, terraforming is well on its way and the aerial view of the Labyrinth of Night is changing accordingly. The frost on the highlands has almost completely vanished, and plant life is spreading through the valleys.

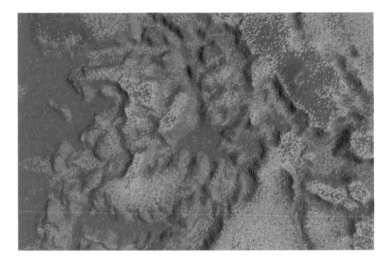

Four centuries after the last time we looked down on the Labyrinth of Night, extensive forests of oak trees cover much of the lower ground – although they are barely visible, except as colour altera-tions, from such a high altitude as this (still one hundred kilo-metres). There is liquid water around but, the atmosphere being still tenuous, much more remains locked up in frozen form. This balance will shift very soon: only a century later (OPPOSITE), in AD2800, new seas are forming and the Labyrinth of Night is beginning to flood, creating islands to which the human inhabitants of Mars have given names nostalgically reminiscent of humankind's cradle world: here you can find Bali, Ceylon, Tahiti, Delos . . . and Avalon.

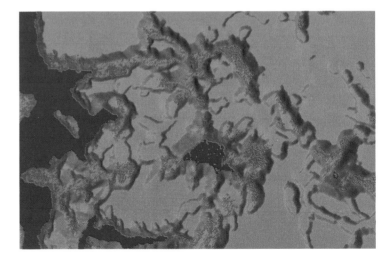

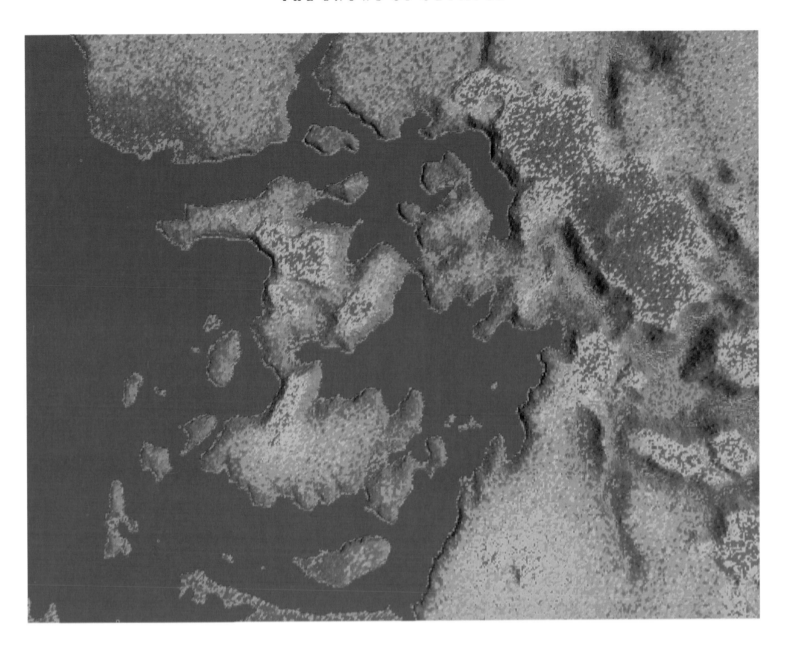

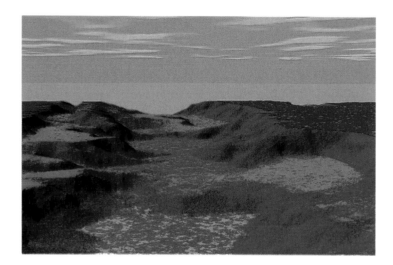

The long narrow canyon Tithonius Chasm (Tithonium Chasma) runs off the eastern end of the Labyrinth of Night (see picture on page 83). We first see it (LEFT) in the very early stages of terraforming, in about the year AD2200. The atmosphere still has its original pink colour, but various coloured lichens, adapted from terrestrial strains, are spreading across the canyon and, as we can see on the far right, beginning to conquer the higher ground. BELOW: The same scene, two centuries later. So far there are few observable differences in the vegetation cover; the big change is in the atmosphere, which has become denser and bluer.

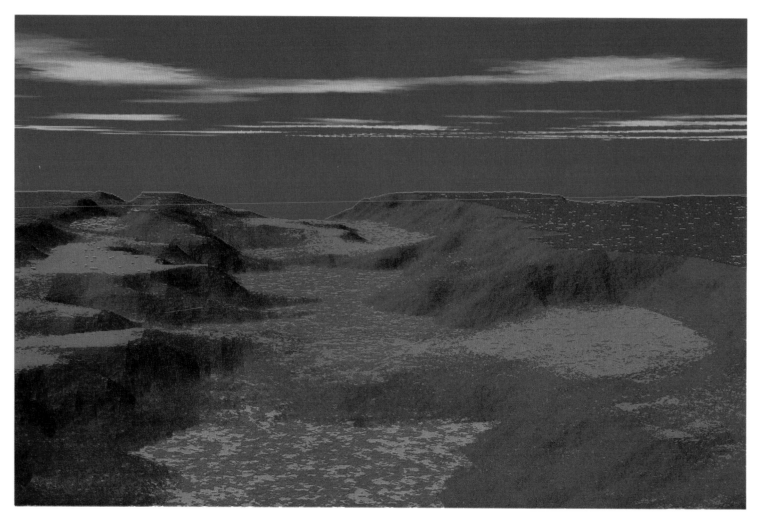

RIGHT: **A further century has passed: it is now AD2500. The shallow lakes that have formed in the valley, like those elsewhere on the partially terraformed Mars, remain frozen most of the year.**
BELOW: **Two hundred years later, and now we can see how profound are the changes that terraforming has wrought. In this once lifeless place, mutated pines are thriving: we can see them climbing the lower slopes of the chasm. At least during the summer, the lakes thaw, so that seasonal vegetation can prosper around their shores.**

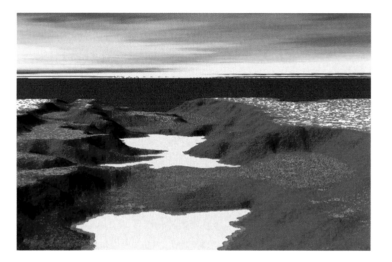

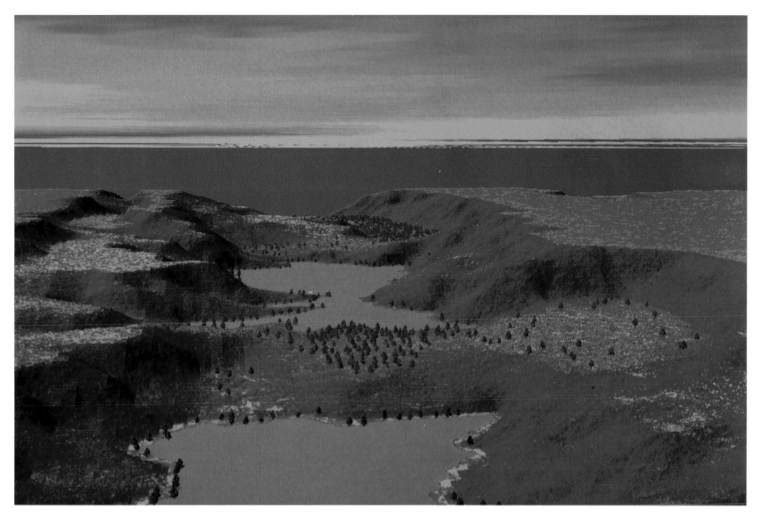

OPPOSITE: **It is all too easy for us to forget, when looking at artists' 'preconstructions' of humankind's future on Mars, that the planet has an atmosphere. Here, perhaps within a couple of hundred years of the start of terraforming, it already makes sense to use parachutes to slow the rate of final descent of unmanned container vessels from orbit. Obviously it will be yet further centuries before conventional parachuting will be feasible – although alert readers will have noticed the hydrogen balloon in the distance beyond the AD2200 Mars base depicted on page 33.** (*Painting by Michael Carroll, reproduced by permission*)

PART III

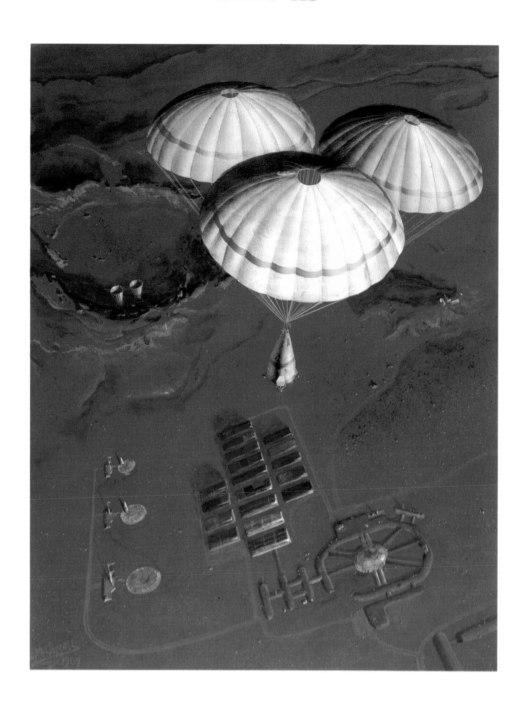

8

The Longest Spring

Tomorrow to fresh woods and pastures new.
John Milton, *Lycidas*

At the climax of the movie *Total Recall* (1990) the life-support system of a Martian colony is sabotaged. In the nick of time, our hero (Arnold Schwarzenegger) discovers a gigantic buried machine built by some vanished race and is able to switch it on. From a standing start it gives Mars a breathable atmosphere in about sixty seconds flat. Ridiculous!

At this point, someone may remind me of Clarke's Third Law: 'Any sufficiently advanced technology is indistinguishable from magic.' But even the most optimistic planetary engineers believe that to replenish the atmosphere of Mars would take not seconds but *centuries* – and more likely millennia.

Converting Mars into a world that is habitable by unprotected humans is a thought experiment on the grand scale, which is perhaps why it has attracted a large number of first-class minds. One of them was the maverick astronomical genius Fritz Zwicky, who in his 1946 Halley Lecture stunned his fellow astronomers by talking about reconstructing the Solar System to make it a more desirable piece of real estate. Freeman Dyson – another certified, card-carrying genius – went into some of the practical details in his aptly named book *Disturbing the Universe* (1979). So did James Lovelock, originator of the controversial Gaia hypothesis, in *The Greening of Mars* (1984, with Michael Allaby).

Creating Mars Mark II (perhaps it should be Mark III, as there may once have been a habitable Mark I) would involve raising the planet's mean surface temperature by about 50°C (80°F) and increasing the density of its atmosphere almost a hundredfold – assuming that half this increase was due to oxygen. The two challenges are not separate, but closely related, as providing an atmosphere of almost any kind would raise the temperature of Mars through the greenhouse effect.

Notwithstanding its brilliance in our night sky, the surface of Mars is fairly dark, reflecting back only about sixteen per cent of the sunlight falling on it. The dazzlingly white polar caps are responsible for most of this, and it has been suggested that coating these areas with black material – a few million tons of soot (carbon), for example – would have the dual effect of raising the mean temperature and releasing the vast quantities of frozen carbon dioxide and water trapped at the poles. Where would we get the carbon? Well, a few billion tons may be orbiting overhead: Phobos is one of the *blackest* bodies in the Solar System, with the reflectivity of coal. However, it would make more sense to obtain carbon from the local carbon-dioxide-bearing minerals (carbonates), releasing much-needed oxygen in the process.

A considerably more attractive – and more environmentally benign – approach would be to increase the level of solar radiation on Mars by the use of orbiting mirrors. As the desirable value would be about twice the present one, the total mirror area would have to be comparable to that of Mars itself – i.e., about ten million square kilometres. Fortunately the reflecting material need be only a few atoms thick, and so we could use the technology made available during the development of solar-sailing spacecraft (see pages 37–8). Indeed, these mirrors might later be engaged in some solar sailing of their own: once they had fulfilled their Martian contracts they could make their leisurely way to parts of the Solar System where they were even more badly needed, such as around the moons of Jupiter.

Warming an entire planet by *artificial* means seems preposterous, but it may be another possibility in the distant future. During the last fifty years – a moment in human history

94

– we have made the millionfold jump from chemical to atomic energy . . . yet the nuclear fission (uranium) reaction, the only one we can currently control, has an efficiency of a miserable 0.1 per cent! Compare that with the few per cent of hydrogen fusion – and the *one hundred per cent* of the matter-antimatter reaction! Clearly, we still have a very long way to go.

In my novel *The Sands of Mars* (1951) I suggested that one way this might be done was to trigger a 'meson resonance reaction' on the moon Phobos, so that it would burn like a tiny sun for 1000 years or so; this new luminary would give the Martian surface about a tenth of the Sun's heat, in due course bringing it up to nearly the same temperature as Earth's. For over forty years I assumed that a 'meson resonance reaction' was nothing more than a science-fiction writer's gobbledegook, but now I am not so sure.

The term 'meson' is used generically for short-lived sub-atomic particles which come in a variety of masses. One of the most important types is the mu-meson, or muon, which is similar to the electron except that it is unstable and 207 times heavier. In 1947 the UK physicist Charles Frank, working on cosmic rays at Bristol University, began to wonder if mesons could be used to catalyze nuclear reactions at relatively low temperatures (i.e., to support 'cold' fusion). Frank's idea came to the attention of an obscure Russian physicist, Andrei Sakharov, who in 1948 wrote a memorandum on the subject entitled 'Passive Mesons'. However, Sakharov was then on the team developing the hydrogen bomb, and his paper was a secret internal report of the Lebedev Institute, so nothing much happened in this area until 1956, by which time both the United States and the USSR had exploded H-bombs. Later that year a team under Luis Alvarez at Berkeley, California, succeeded in creating muon fusion on a limited scale and, as Alvarez wrote afterwards, had a 'short but exhilarating experience when we thought we had solved all of the fuel problems of mankind for the rest of time'. Unfortunately, their discovery soon appeared to be a false hope; muons do not live long enough to run a chain reaction. But the 'cold' fusion dream has not died – very much to the contrary. Even as I write, teams of scientists in many countries are working towards that goal: if they succeed, the Age of Fossil Fuels may be over.

None of this proves, of course, that even an advanced future science could turn a small body like Phobos into a stable mini-sun; but at least the idea has some tenuous basis in genuine physics. A more promising candidate for starmaking might be Jupiter, which has often been called 'a star that failed'. Perhaps a few strategically placed black holes might do the trick – as suggested in *2010: Odyssey Two* (1980) – although of course this would not much affect distant Mars.

Let us assume, then, that by some means or other Mars has been given an equable temperature. That would not be much of an improvement if the atmosphere were still only one-hundredth as dense as that at the top of Everest and water were virtually nonexistent. Megatons – gigatons – of nitrogen, oxygen and hydrogen would have to be found, somewhere. If they once existed in quantity on Mars, could they still be there?

Undoubtedly there are vast quantities of frozen water and carbon dioxide trapped in the polar caps, but even the release of all of it would go only a small way to solving the problem. Possibly there may be lost Martian oceans in the form of permafrost a few metres below the surface of much of the planet. We simply do not know: looking for such deposits will be the first order of business for future explorers, human and robot.

It has also been suggested that much of the planet's carbon and oxygen may, over geological periods of time, have become locked up in minerals such as calcite ($CaCO_3$). Releasing carbon dioxide (CO_2) from this on a global scale would require staggering amounts of energy – the equivalent of tens of *millions* of high-yield nuclear bombs. The notion of 'thermo-nuclear mining' to release volatile materials from the Martian crust has been only half-seriously proposed: it is not one that is likely to arouse much enthusiasm among the colonists.

So perhaps we must look elsewhere. We know that space is full of ice; frozen water, together with many useful carbon compounds, may be a principal component of many comets and some of the satellites of the outer planets. Only a modest amount of rocket thrust, applied at the appropriate time and place, could nudge a suitable comet into a trajectory that would impact Mars.

This may sound as bad for the local environment as thermo-nuclear mining. However, a small comet, overtaking Mars at a low relative velocity, would break up in the atmosphere and – hopefully – descend as a harmless shower of ice. In fact, according to a recent controversial theory, this is happening to the Earth all the time, as hundreds of large 'snowballs' enter our atmosphere every day! It has even been suggested that our oceans originally had such an extraterrestrial origin.

*

The establishment of scientific bases on Mars could be well under way by the middle of the twenty-first century, and by its end there may even be small autonomous settlements on the planet. But it might seem that large-scale terraforming, if possible at all, would take thousands – perhaps tens of thousands – of years.

This is probably true if one thinks in terms of current technologies for manipulating bulk matter. But we are now on the verge of a revolution that will do for manufacturing processes what the microchip has done for computing. It involves two key elements: von Neumann machines and nanotechnology.

A von Neumann machine* is any device – perhaps it would be better to call it a system – which can collect energy and material from its surrounding environment and use them to manufacture a working (though seldom identical) copy of itself. Such machines are extremely common; you will see one if you look in your mirror. Nature invented von Neumann machines billions of years ago, the first and still the most successful models being bacteria. While living von Neumann machines (like yourself) have become considerably more complex since then, the basic principle is unchanged. That principle will soon be applied to mechanical, as opposed to biological, systems to produce something that sounds like a classic science-fiction nightmare, the self-replicating robot. However, these 'robots' will be machines specially designed for an endless variety of tasks, and many of them will be too small to be visible to the naked eye. This will be made possible through the submicro-engineering techniques which now allow us to manipulate single atoms. We will be able to build machines on the nanometre (billionth of a metre) scale – hence the term 'nanotechnology' – to carry out almost any conceivable task, and at unprecedented speeds, thanks to their self-reproducing ability. Chemical engineering, agriculture, mining and indeed almost every type of industrial operation will be transformed. In fact, the first two of the above enterprises have employed von Neumann machines for thousands of years. The benign bacteria which create cheese and wine, or those which trap nitrogen when the farmer rotates his crops, are self-replicating chemical factories. You need only a spoonful of them to get started; then you can be in business for ever, on any scale you wish, as they happily multiply and work for you.

What makes the potential of von Neumann machines so awesome is their ability to multiply exponentially – assuming, of course, that the necessary supply of raw materials is available. Suppose the time required to make a copy is one hour; then, with the striking of the clock marking each generation, the numbers increase in the geometric sequence 2, 4, 8, 16, 32, 64, 128, 256 . . . so that by the end of the tenth hour there are 1024 copies, after twenty hours a million, after thirty hours a billion – need I go on? Were it not for the limiting speed of light, in a few weeks the whole visible Universe would be converted . . .

The application to terraforming should now be clear: if the Moon were a big ball of milk, a spoonful of the right enzyme could turn it into the traditional green cheese between new and full. Many years ago I came across a slightly more practicable but still quite large-scale example of – literally – terraforming. The story may be apocryphal but no matter – it illustrates the point perfectly.

Once upon a time there was a large area of useless and frequently flooded marshland in a remote part of Canada. The local authorities wished to develop it for agricultural purposes. However, to have reclaimed it by bulldozers and earth-moving machinery would have cost millions and taken years. Then a local wildlife expert pointed out that the job could be done for nothing – assuming there was no particular hurry. He suggested importing some readily available von Neumann machines: beavers. Given a few decades, they would remake the landscape – and they did.

The von Neumann machines which remake Mars and perhaps much of the Solar System will have to be programmed with far greater skills, and be made of considerably tougher materials,

*The name honours the Hungarian–US mathematician John von Neumann (1903–1957), who first worked out the principles in connection with his work on electronic computers.

OPPOSITE: *Ice Asteroids for Mars*, **by David A. Hardy. We are still not certain how much water may be hidden in frozen form beneath the Martian desert, nor how easily the settlers will be able to extract it in the initial stages of terraforming. One surprisingly plausible way of ameliorating water shortages would be to import some of the huge quantities of ice floating free in the asteroid belt and among the moons and rings of the giant planets. The areas of impact of these huge blocks of ice would have to be carefully chosen, of course, so that the settlers' lives would not be endangered by, for example, the consequential seismic upheavals; however, the impacts themselves would have a side-effect of creating water-clouds in the atmosphere and thus, in a crude way, assist the initiation of terraforming.** (*Reproduced by permission of David A. Hardy*)

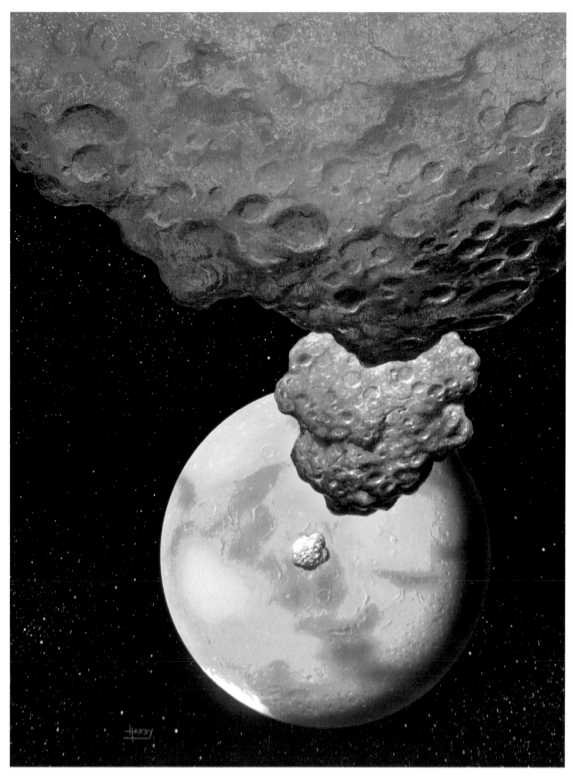

than any that have so far existed on this planet. Here, roughly in chronological sequence, are some of the tasks they might have to perform:

○ visit low-gravity asteroids and satellites to survey them for raw materials;
○ construct solar sails to provide the basis for a fuelless interplanetary transport system;
○ mine suitable comets and satellites for ice and for carbon compounds;
○ ferry (or catapult) this material to the places where it is needed (Mars, the Moon, Venus . . .);
○ continue the operation as long as necessary.

It should be emphasized that, apart from the cost of the first von Neumann machine, there would be no further expense and the entire operation could proceed without human intervention – though occasional human supervision would certainly be desirable. Even if that first machine cost a trillion dollars – as it well might – all the rest, from the second to infinity, would cost nothing.

Freeman Dyson, in *Disturbing the Universe* (1979), gives a possible scenario for the terraforming of Mars using material from Saturn's moon Enceladus – which, judging by its density, is largely ice:

The experiment begins with a rocket, carrying a small but highly sophisticated payload launched from Earth . . . The payload contains an automaton capable of reproducing itself out of the materials available on Enceladus, using as energy source the feeble light of the far-distant Sun. The automaton is programmed to produce progeny that are miniature solar sailboats, each carrying a wide, thin sail with which it can navigate in space . . . Each sailboat carries into space a small block of ice from Enceladus. The sole purpose of the sailboats is to deliver their cargo of ice safely to Mars . . . A few years later, the nighttime sky of Mars begins to glow bright with an incessant sparkle of small meteors. The infall continues day and night . . . soft breezes blow over the land, and slowly warmth penetrates into the frozen ground. A little later, it rains on Mars for the first time in a billion years. It does not take long for oceans to begin to grow. There is enough ice on Enceladus to keep the Martian climate warm for ten thousand years and to make the Martian deserts bloom . . .

Dyson is careful to describe this vision of the future as a thought experiment, and it is more than likely that, by the time we attempt such grandiose schemes, we will possess far more powerful technologies than those outlined in his scenario. For example, we may obtain complete mastery of the forces holding the atomic nucleus together and thus achieve the alchemists' dream of transmutation; however, we would not waste such powers on anything so trivial as turning lead into gold but instead use them on barren worlds to create such *really* valuable elements as oxygen, hydrogen, carbon, nitrogen and phosphorus – the essential building blocks of life itself.

In a 1991 paper in the UK science journal *Nature*, 'Making Mars Habitable',* the authors describe how Mars might be made capable of supporting genetically modified plants and bacteria; then, much later, animals. The technologies suggested include orbiting mirrors, spraying the polar caps with absorbing material, and the injection of chlorofluorine compounds into the atmosphere to accelerate the greenhouse effect. The timescales suggested vary from a few centuries to 100,000 years, depending upon the availability of local materials.

By one means or another, in the centuries that lie ahead, the long, slow spring will come to Mars.

*By Christopher P. McKay, Owen B. Toon, James F. Kasting; vol 352, pp 489–96, 8 August 1991.

'Disneymars'

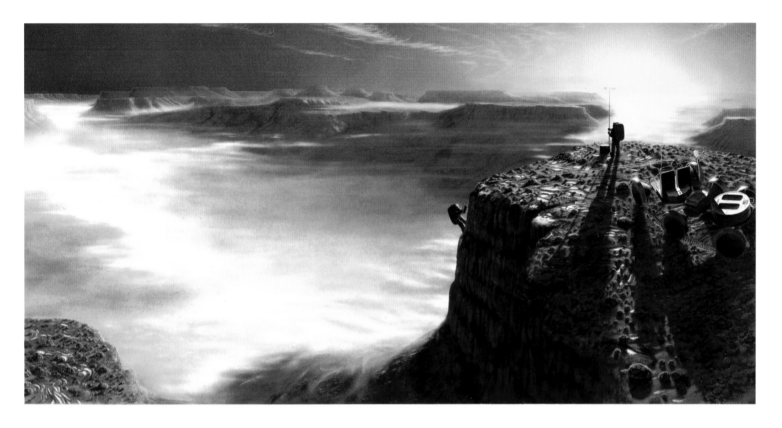

In my novel The Hammer of God *(1993) I described how visitors to 'Disneymars' might have a preview of their own future:*

The final exhibit was almost old-fashioned in its simplicity, and none the less effective. They sat in near-darkness behind a picture-window, looking down upon a sea of mist, while the distant Sun came up behind them.

'Mariner Valley – the Labyrinth of Night, as it is today,' said a soft voice above a background of gentle music.

The mist dissolved beneath the rising Sun; it was no more than the thinnest of vapours. And there was the vast expanse of canyons and cliffs of the mightiest valley in the Solar System, sharp and clear out to the horizon, with none of the softening by distance that gave a sense of perspective to similar views in the far smaller Grand Canyon of Western America.

Most of the outdoor sports and recreations that we take for granted will have to be severely adapted if the colonists are to enjoy them on Mars – but, by contrast, mountaineering and rock-climbing will become staple practices for those whose jobs require them to get from one place to another at short notice and with the minimum of fuss, like these two maintenance experts checking a mountaintop installation. (*Painting by Pat Rawlings, reproduced by permission*)

It was austerely beautiful, with its reds and ochres and crimsons, not so much hostile to life as utterly indifferent to it. The eye looked in vain for the slightest hint of blue or green.

The Sun dashed swiftly across the sky, the shadows flowed like tides of ink over the canyon floors. Night fell; the stars flashed out briefly, and were banished by another dawn.

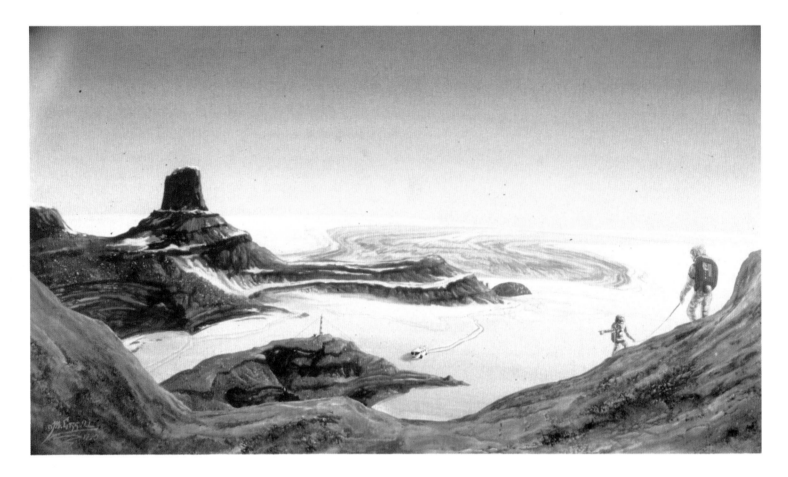

Nothing had changed – or had it? Was the far horizon no longer so sharp-edged?

Another 'day', and there could be no doubt. The harsh contours of the terrain were becoming softened; distant cliffs and scars were no longer so sharply defined. Mars was changing . . .

The days – weeks – months – perhaps they were really decades – flickered past. And now the changes were dramatic.

The faint salmon hue of the sky had given way to a pale blue, and at last real clouds were forming – not tenuous mists that vanished with the dawn. And down on the floor of the canyon, patches of green weř spreading where once there had been only barren rock. There were no trees as yet, but lichens and mosses were preparing the way.

Suddenly, magically, there were pools of water – lying calm and unruffled in the Sun, not flashing instantly into vapour as they would on Mars today. As the vision of the future unfolded,

Whatever the degree of terraforming that has taken place, the south polar region of Mars, like that of our own planet, will almost certainly forever remain a hostile place – and thus a focus for the diehard Scotts and Nansens of future generations . . . (*Painting by Pat Rawlings, reproduced by permission*)

the pools became lakes, and merged into a river. Trees sprouted abruptly along its banks: to Robert Singh's Earth-conditioned eyes, their trunks appeared so slender that he could not believe they were more than a dozen metres tall. In reality – if one could call this reality! – they would probably out-top the tallest redwood: 100m, at a minimum, in this low gravity.

Now the viewpoint changed; they were flying eastwards along Mariner Valley, out through the Chasm of the Dawn, and southwards to the great plain of Hellas, the lowlands of Mars. It was land no longer.

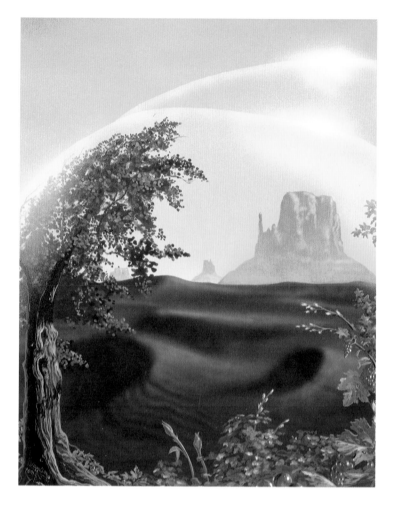

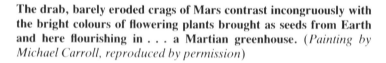

The drab, barely eroded crags of Mars contrast incongruously with the bright colours of flowering plants brought as seeds from Earth and here flourishing in . . . a Martian greenhouse. (*Painting by Michael Carroll, reproduced by permission*)

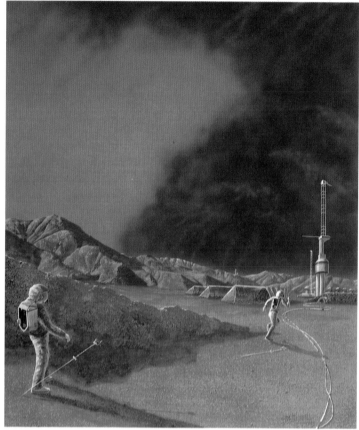

Long after humankind has established itself on Mars, and even with terraforming several centuries under way, one peril will remain: dust-storms. Today a full-blown Martian dust-storm can obscure significant portions of the planet's disc; to the early generations of colonists it could spell terminal catastrophe. (*Painting by Michael Carroll, reproduced by permission*)

. . . The voyage into the future ended with a glimpse of the planet Mars from space – how many centuries or millennia hence? – its poles no longer crowned with caps of frozen carbon dioxide, as sunlight beamed down from 100km-wide orbiting mirrors ended their age-long winter. The image faded, to be replaced by the words SPRING, 2500. I wonder – I hope so, though I shall never know, thought Robert Singh as they walked out in silence. Even Mirelle seemed unusually subdued, as if trying to disentangle the real from the imaginary in what she had seen.

As they were walking through the airlock to the pressurized marscar that had brought them from the hotel, the Exhibition produced one final surprise. There was a roll of distant thunder – a sound that only Robert Singh had ever heard in reality – and Mirelle gave a little shriek as a shower of fine droplets fell upon them from an overhead sprinkler.

'The last rain on Mars was three billion years ago – and it brought no life to the lands on which it fell.

'Next time, it will be different. Goodbye, and thank you for coming . . .'

9

Concerning Ends and Means

Let us stand back and take the longer view, to try and get these ideas in perspective.

There are many, even among those who think that terraforming is quite possible, who believe that it should not be attempted. I must confess that I have a considerable sympathy for this view: one of my favourite quotations is Thoreau's 'In wildness is the preservation of the world'. I would not like to see all of the magnificent Martian wildness – or wilderness – tamed and turned into parkland. (For a brilliant dramatization of this future conflict, giving a fair treatment to both points of view, see Kim Stanley Robinson's *Red Mars* [1992].)

A recent issue of the *Journal of the British Interplanetary Society* (vol 42 no 12, December 1989) was devoted to terraforming. One member, Enrico Coffey, asked:

Could terraforming another world ever be justified? Is it a laudable aim or a terrible folly? . . . What if it was completely disastrous? In a sense, man has long conducted an uncontrolled experiment in terraforming a planet and the verdict is already coming in: global climatic change (such as worldwide warming, and greatly exacerbated tempests); colossal devastation of natural habitats, worsened by burgeoning population; human-induced soil erosion; likely increased melting of icecaps and consequent raised sea-level; polluted food and water supplies; and so on. The cause of this, for both political and economic reasons, is a persistent ignoring of the full consequences of technological activities. Are we, therefore, to give up on our own world, and instead export out into the Universe that very same ideology which is on the verge of destroying our home planet?

At the root of the problem lies an unacknowledged ideology: the Western paradigm, whose ancient imperative (supposedly divinely inspired) is that the world and its denizens are for us to do with as we wish, for us to dominate. It prevents us from living in harmony with the world, hence with the Universe. Likewise, a terraformed world would be essentially a controlled environment in which all that was

wild, exotic, hostile and dangerous would have been eliminated. We would create only an impoverished world.

There is also the argument, first advocated by J. D. Bernal in what has often been called the best book about the future ever written, *The World, the Flesh and the Devil* (1929), that planets are not the right place to live, anyway. Our ultimate home will be space, in the weightless environment of artificial worlds that can be created nearer to our hearts' desire. More recently, the late Gerard O'Neill promoted the idea in his book *The High Frontier* (1977); and, perhaps biased by my scuba-diving experiences, I too have argued that we will not be really happy until we can escape from gravity. We are exiles here on dry land, in transit between the ocean of water in which we were born and the ocean of space where most of history will run its course.

Perhaps. I have no doubt that space colonies will be built, some of enormous size. But there is a great deal to be said for a planetary environment, and gravity is not all bad. Because it has such enormous inertia, a planet is a fail-safe, automatically correcting system: it is not easy to wreck it, though sometimes we seem to be doing our best here on Earth. In comparison, space colonies appear fragile constructions with few back-ups – disasters waiting to happen.

In 1950, at the exact midpoint of the century, and seven years before the Space Age opened, I concluded my first book on astronautics, *Interplanetary Flight: An Introduction to Astronautics*, with words which are even more relevant today:

No one can ever foresee what role a new land may play in history; and we are considering now not merely new countries, or even continents – but worlds.

But the important consequences of spaceflight, and the main reasons for its accomplishment, are intangible, and to understand them we must look not to the future but to the past. Although man has occupied the greater part of the habitable globe for thousands of years, until only five centuries ago he lived – psychologically – not in one world but in many. Each of the great cultures in the belt from the UK to Japan was insulated from its neighbours by geography or deliberate choice: each was convinced that it alone represented the flower of civilization, and that all else was barbarism.

The 'unification of the world', to use Toynbee's somewhat optimistic phrase, became possible only when the sailing ship and the arts of navigation were developed sufficiently to replace the difficult overland routes by the easier sea-passages. The result was the great age of exploration whose physical climax was the discovery of the Americas, and whose supreme intellectual achievement was the liberation of the human spirit. Perhaps no better symbol of the questing mind of Renaissance man could be found than the lonely ship sailing steadfastly towards new horizons, until east and west had merged at last and the circumnavigation of the globe had been achieved.

First by land, then by sea, man grew to know his planet; but its final conquest was to lie in a third element, and by means beyond the imagination of almost all men who had ever lived before the twentieth century. The swiftness with which mankind has lifted its commerce and its wars into the air has surpassed the wildest fantasy. Now indeed we have fulfilled the poet's dream and can 'ride secure the cruel sky'. Through this mastery the last unknown lands have been opened up: over the road along which Alexander burnt out his life, the businessmen and civil servants now pass in comfort in a matter of hours.

The victory has been complete, yet in the winning it has turned to ashes. Every age but ours has had its El Dorado, its Happy Isles, or its North-West Passage to lure the adventurous into the unknown. A lifetime ago men could still dream of what might lie at the poles – but now the North Pole is the crossroads of the world. We may try to console ourselves with the thought that, even if Earth has no new horizons, there are no bounds to the endless frontier of science. Yet it may be doubted if this is enough, for only very sophisticated minds are satisfied with purely intellectual adventures.

The importance of exploration does not lie merely in the opportunities it gives to the adolescent (but not to be despised) desires for excitement and variety. It is no mere accident that the age of Columbus was also the age of Leonardo, or that Sir Walter Raleigh was a contemporary of Shakespeare and Galileo. 'In human records,' wrote the

anthropologist J. D. Unwin, 'there is no trace of any display of productive energy which has not been preceded by a display of expansive energy.' And, today, all possibility of expansion on Earth itself has practically ceased.

The thought is a sombre one. Even if it survives the hazards of war, our culture is proceeding under a momentum which must be exhausted in the foreseeable future. [Jean Henri] Fabre once described how he linked the two ends of a chain of marching caterpillars so that they circled endlessly in a closed loop. Even if we avoid all other disasters, this would appear a fitting symbol of humanity's eventual fate when the impetus of the last few centuries has reached its peak and died away. For a closed culture, though it may endure for centuries, is inherently unstable. It may decay quietly and crumble into ruin, or it may be disrupted violently by internal conflicts. Space travel is a necessary, though not in itself a sufficient, way of escape from this predicament.

It is now 400 years since Copernicus destroyed medieval cosmology and dethroned the Earth from the centre of creation. Shattering though the repercussions of that fall were in the fields of science and philosophy, they scarcely touched the ordinary man. To him this planet is still the whole of the Universe; he knows that other worlds exist, but the knowledge does not affect his life and therefore has little real meaning to him.

All this will be changed before the twentieth century draws to its end. Into a few decades may be compressed more profound alterations in our world picture than occurred during the whole of the Renaissance and the Age of Discovery that followed. To our children the Moon may become what the Americas were 400 years ago – a world of unknown danger, promise and opportunity. No longer will Mars and Venus be merely the names of wandering lights seldom glimpsed by the dwellers in cities. They will be more familiar than ever they were to those eastern watchers who first marked their movements, for they will be the new frontiers of the human mind.

Those new frontiers are urgently needed. The crossing of space – even the mere belief in its possibility – may do much to reduce the tensions of our age by turning men's minds outwards and away from their tribal conflicts. It may well be that only by acquiring this new sense of boundless frontiers will the world break free from the ancient cycle of war and peace. One wonders how even the most stubborn of nationalisms will survive when men have seen the Earth as a pale crescent dwindling against the stars, until at last they look for it in vain.

No doubt there are many who, while agreeing that these things are possible, will shrink from them in horror, hoping that they will never come to pass. They remember Pascal's terror of the silent spaces between the stars, and are overwhelmed by the nightmare immensities which Victorian astronomers were so fond of evoking. Such an outlook is somewhat naïve, for the meaningless millions of miles between the Sun and its outermost planets are no more, and no less, impressive than the vertiginous gulf lying between the electron and the atomic nucleus. Mere distance is nothing: only the time that is needed to span it has any meaning. A spaceship which can reach the Moon at all would require less time for the journey than a stagecoach once took to travel the length of England. When the atomic drive is reasonably efficient, the nearer planets would be only a few weeks from Earth, and so will seem scarcely more remote that are the antipodes today.

It is fascinating, however premature, to try to imagine the pattern of events when the Solar System is opened up to mankind. In the footsteps of the first explorers will follow the scientists and engineers, shaping strange environments with technologies as yet unborn. Later will come the colonists, laying the foundations of cultures which in time may surpass those of the mother world. The torch of civilization has dropped from failing fingers too often before for us to imagine that it will never be handed on again.

We must not let our pride in our achievements blind us to the lessons of history. Over the first cities of mankind, the desert sands now lie centuries deep. Could the builders of Ur and Babylon – once the wonders of the world – have pictured London or New York? Nor can we imagine the citadels that our descendants may one day build beneath the blistering Sun of Mercury, or under the stars of the cold Plutonian wastes. And beyond the planets, though ages still ahead of us in time, lies the unknown and infinite promise of the stellar Universe.

There will, it is true, be danger in space, as there has always been on the oceans or in the air. Some of these dangers we may guess: others we shall not know until we meet them. Nature is no friend of man's, and the most that he can hope for is her neutrality. But if he meets destruction, it will be at his own hands and according to a familiar pattern.

The dream of flight was one of the noblest, and one of the most disinterested, of all man's aspirations. Yet it led in the end to that silver Superfortress driving in passionless beauty through August skies towards the city whose name it was to sear into the conscience of the world.

That is the danger, the dark thundercloud that threatens the promise of the dawn. The rocket has already been the instrument of evil, and may be so again. But there is no way back into the past: the choice, as Wells once said, is the Universe – or nothing. Though men and civilizations may yearn for rest, for the dream of the lotus-eaters, that is a desire that merges imperceptibly into death. The challenge of the great spaces between the worlds is a stupendous one; but, if we fail to meet it, the story of our race will be drawing to its close. Humanity will have turned its back upon the still untrodden heights and will be descending the long slope that stretches, across a thousand million years of time, down to the shores of the primeval sea.

Appendix 1

Extract from *The Mars Project: Journeys Beyond the Cold War*
by Senator Spark Matsunaga

. . . I decided to contact Dr Arthur C. Clarke, my nomination for Space Age man for all seasons. When he wasn't guiding our imaginations to new celestial worlds, Clarke applied his considerable scientific acumen to translating his visions into practical reality. In a sense, the Space Age began when, shortly after World War II, Arthur Clarke conceptualized the first communications satellite. I had read his essays on the unifying powers of Space Age technology, in which he moved a step beyond Marshall McLuhan's global village and postulated a global family. But I was especially drawn to his most recent novel, *2010: Odyssey Two* [1982], the sequel to his epic *2001: A Space Odyssey* [1968], telling the story of a joint US–USSR mission to Jupiter.

Dr Clarke lived halfway around the world, in the island nation of Sri Lanka, off the coast of India. Through his agent in New York, Russell Galen, I obtained his address. Late one night at the office, as I was writing to Clarke to ask him for a letter of support, I happened to glance over at the television set across from my desk, with its attached video cassette recorder, and it occurred to me: Clarke was a genius at imaginative presentation – why not invite him to submit his testimony on a videotape?

His reply came by telephone from Sri Lanka. He loved the idea. He had his own private filming studio. He would put his other work aside and begin at once.

The Clarke videotape arrived by courier on Monday, September 10, barely three days before the hearing. But the videotape was made on the European PAL system, and I couldn't find a film laboratory in Washington that could convert it to the US system in time for the hearing. When Clarke learned by phone of my difficulty he activated his own private global communications network. The next thing I knew, the videotape was being rushed to a laboratory in New York, converted, and returned to my office the next morning. Never to my knowledge had a witness worked harder, at his own considerable expense, to deliver testimony at a Congressional hearing.

I previewed the videotape on Wednesday evening in the Senate recording studio. It ran for fifteen minutes – precisely the length requested – and it was superb. It opened like a movie, with title and credits. I had requested Clarke's views on an international Mars mission, and he replied with:

A MARTIAN ODYSSEY
VIDEO PRESENTATION TO THE COMMITTEE ON
FOREIGN RELATIONS
UNITED STATES SENATE
1984 September 13

Arthur Clarke appeared on the screen, seated at a desk in his book-lined study in Sri Lanka, a trim, balding gentleman wearing a gray suit, light-blue shirt, and royal-blue tie, relaxed, almost bemused at being called upon to explain what seemed to him so obvious. With a true director's eye, he broke up his lecture by shifting camera angles, occasionally using personal mementos to illustrate a point – a photograph with Soviet cosmonaut Alexei Leonov, an inscribed portrait of US astronaut Tom Stafford.

Clarke left no doubt how he felt about the Soviet regime. Not only had he dedicated *2010* to Leonov and Andrei Sakharov, but the seven Russian crew members in the novel were named after Soviet dissidents. 'My Moscow friend and editor failed to spot these curious coincidences,' Clarke recounted, 'and has accordingly lost his job.'

Clarke understood the Cold War, and he also understood the stupidity and futility of carrying it into the cosmos. With his usual foresight, he had issued his first warnings against that prospect in the 1940s. Space weapons were incompatible with any creative vision of our future in space. He called them 'technological obscenities'. 'Let us now talk about technological decency,' Clarke said:

Fifteen years ago at the Cape, when we had finished cheering the first men on their way to the Moon, I saw the Vice-President of the United States turn to Walter Cronkite and say that we could put a man on Mars by the end of the century – and 'we should do it . . . because the people want something to look forward to as an exciting objective.' That sentence echoes a much more ancient saying that might well serve as a motto for your Committee: 'Without vision, the people perish.'

Could we put a man on Mars by the end of the century – now only one year further away than the launch of *Apollo* 11? Let me give the views of a man who, perhaps better than anyone, can answer that question.

With appropriate serendipity, Dr Tom Paine, NASA Administrator for the critical years 1968–1970, has just sent me the paper 'A Timeline for Martian Pioneers' he delivered at the University of Colorado in July. Here is his prediction for the period beginning 1995 – repeat, 1995: 'The decade opens with a triumphant Soviet expedition to Mars, including docking scenes at Phobos with spectacular extra-vehicular activities . . . that dominate TV. The President of the United States receives a Golden Fleece from an elderly senator for relinquishing the United States' scientific pre-eminence to the Soviet Union. In response, he orders the Vice-President to overhaul the US space program; she begins by firing the NASA Administrator for lack of boldness . . .'

Dr Paine has his tongue in his cheek, of course, but he is also deadly serious. When it is ready, the USSR will go to Mars. Why are its cosmonauts making space endurance records with times approaching those required for the Earth–Mars round trip? You don't need *that* capability for missions this side of the Moon!

Sooner than they imagine, Americans will have to ask themselves: 'Do we stand aside, when the Soviet Union heads for Mars? Do we go it alone? Or do we go with them?'

I admit my bias – indeed, my interest – in this area. As you doubtless know, the novel *2010: Odyssey Two* describes a joint US–USSR mission – though to Jupiter, not Mars!

The novel is dedicated to Cosmonaut General Alexei Leonov, the first man to walk in space, and commander of the *Apollo–Soyuz* rendezvous. He was delighted to know that the ship is named after him: 'Then it will be a good ship!' he exclaimed, when I told him this, in his apartment at 'Star Village'.

You may not remember that the *Apollo–Soyuz* mission was itself directly inspired by a Hollywood movie, *Marooned* [1969]. Frankly, one of my purposes in writing *2010* was to start people thinking seriously again about such cooperation.

I am not so naïve as to imagine that this could be achieved without excruciating difficulty, and major changes in the present political climate . . . Most of those changes will have to be made in Moscow, and may have to await the long-overdue extinction of the Kremlin dinosaurs . . .

. . . What we must do is strengthen and extend any existing space agreements. For example, the combined US–USSR–Canadian–French 'Search and Rescue' satellite (SARSAT) has already saved scores of lives, on the high seas and in the Arctic. If the public knew more about it, there would be a demand for more programs of this kind . . .

. . . Though unmanned space missions are essential and often highly cost-effective, they do not fire the imagination. And, contrary to what some scientists may have told you, in the long run it is the *manned* missions that will be the more important. Unfortunately, no one can predict whether that run will last for centuries, or mere decades. Almost certainly it will exceed the attention span of even the most enlightened Administration.

I have just been listening to an historic and inspiring sound from the past – the applause of Congress as President Kennedy cried: 'We choose to go to the Moon!' One day the United States will return to the Moon. That will be exciting and important; but it will no longer be pioneering. The Moon, though an essential stepping-stone to space, is only the offshore island of Earth. But Mars – a planet as large as our own, in terms of land area, is the first of the New Worlds.

Only eight years from now it will be exactly half a millennium since three tiny ships sailed forth from Spain, to change the history of our species. And three is about right for the smallest practical Mars expedition – one unmanned cargo vessel, and two manned ships, either able to carry both crews in an emergency. The cost would be less than that proposed merely for *research* into anti-ICBM systems – let alone the bill for their actual deployment, which would be orders of magnitude greater. Even those who think that such expenditure is necessary will surely deplore such a tragic diversion of resources.

So is it absurdly optimistic to hope that, by Columbus Day 1992, the United States and the Soviet Union will have emerged from their long winter of sterile confrontation? That would be none too soon to start talking seriously about mankind's next, and greatest, adventure.

When we said goodbye in 'Star Village', Alexei Leonov – who is a very good artist – gave me a copy of his book *Life Among the Stars*. In it are the sketches he made during the *Apollo–Soyuz* mission, including excellent likenesses of his US colleagues. The portrait of Tom Stafford is autographed as follows: 'To my dear friend Alexei Leonov – many thanks for your friendship and wonderful cooperation – we have opened a new era in the history of man. Tom Stafford, 18 July 1975.'

General Stafford – over to you.

Appendix 2

So You're Going to Mars?

Almost exactly forty years ago, long before the Mariners *and* Vikings *had given us a glimpse of the real Mars – in fact, five years before the Space Age had even opened! – the far-sighted editor of* Holiday Magazine *asked me to write an article* about the planet's tourist possibilities. On re-reading it today I find, to my considerable surprise, that most of it is still perfectly valid – though, I fear, overoptimistic about the possibilities of indigenous Martian life, and the density of the atmosphere. Apart from that, I believe it could stand reprinting for a few centuries; afterwards, it may serve as a reminder of the virgin planet – before terraforming really got under way.*

So you're going to Mars? That's still quite an adventure – though I suppose that in another ten years no one will think twice about it. Sometimes it's hard to remember that the first ships reached Mars scarcely more than half a century ago and that our colony on the planet is less than thirty years old. (By the way, don't use *that* word when you get there. Base, settlement, or whatever you like – but not colony, unless you want to hear the ice tinkling all around you.)

I suppose you've read all the forms and tourist literature they gave you at the Department of Extraterrestrial Affairs. But there's a lot you won't learn just by reading, so here are some pointers and background information that may make your trip more enjoyable. I won't say it's right up to date – things change so rapidly, and it's a year since I got back from Mars myself – but on the whole you'll find it pretty reliable.

Presumably you're going just for curiosity and excitement – because you want to see what life is like out on the new frontier. It's only fair, therefore, to point out that most of your fellow passengers will be engineers, scientists or administrators travelling to Mars – some of them not for the first time – because they've got a job of work to do. So whatever your achievements here on Earth, it's advisable not to talk too much about them, as you'll be among people who've had to tackle much tougher propositions. I won't say that you'll find them boastful: it's simply that they've got a lot to be proud of, and they don't mind who knows it.

If you haven't booked your passage yet, remember that the cost of the ticket varies considerably according to the relative positions of Mars and Earth. That's a complication we don't have to worry about when we're travelling from country to country on our own globe, but Mars can be six times farther away at one time than at another. Oddly enough, the shortest trips are the most expensive since they involve the greatest changes of speed as you hop from one orbit to the other. And in space, speed, not distance, is what costs money.

Incidentally, I'd like to know how you've managed it. I believe the cheapest round trip comes to about thirty thousand Terradollars, and unless the firm is backing you or you've got a very elastic expense account – Oh, all right, if you don't want to talk about it . . .

I take it you're OK on the medical side. That examination isn't for fun, nor is it intended to scare anyone off. The physical strain involved in spaceflight is negligible – but you'll be spending at least two months on the trip, and it would be a pity if your teeth or your appendix started to misbehave. See what I mean?

You're probably wondering how you can possibly manage on the weight allowance you've got. Well, it can be done. The first thing to remember is that you don't need to take any suits. There's no weather inside a spaceship; the temperature never varies more than a couple of degrees over the whole trip, and

*Originally published in *Holiday Magazine*, March 1953, under the title 'A Journey to Mars'.

it's held at a fairly high value so that all you'll want is an ultra-lightweight tropical kit. When you get to Mars you'll buy what you need there and dump it when you return. The great thing to remember is only carry the stuff you actually need *on the trip*. I strongly advise you to buy one of the complete travel kits – they're expensive, but will save you money in excess baggage charges.

Take a camera by all means – there's a chance of some unforgettable shots as you leave Earth and when you approach Mars. But there's nothing to photograph on the voyage itself, and I'd advise you to take all your pictures on the outward trip. You can sell a good camera on Mars for five times its price here – and save yourself the cost of freighting it home. They don't mention *that* in the official handouts.

Now that we've brought up the subject of money, I'd better remind you that the Martian economy is quite different from all those on Earth. Down here, it doesn't cost you anything to breathe, even though you've got to pay to eat. But on Mars the very air has to be synthesized – they break down the oxides in the ground to do this – so every time you fill your lungs someone has to foot the bill. Food production is planned in the same way – each of the cities, remember, is a carefully balanced ecological system, like a well organized aquarium. No parasites can be allowed, so everyone has to pay a basic tax which entitles them to air, food and the shelter of the domes. The tax varies from city to city, but averages about ten Terradollars a day. Since everyone earns at least twenty times as much as this, they can all afford to go on breathing.

You'll have to pay this tax, of course, and you'll find it rather hard to spend much more money than this. Once the basic necessities of life are taken care of, there aren't many luxuries on Mars. When they've got used to the idea of having tourists around, no doubt they'll get organized, but as things are now you'll find that most reasonable requests won't cost you any-thing. However, I should make arrangements to transfer a substantial credit balance to the Bank of Mars – if you've still got anything left.

So much for the preliminaries; now some points about the trip itself. The ferry rocket will probably leave from the New Guinea field, which is about two miles above sea-level on the top of the Orange Range. People sometimes wonder why they chose such an out-of-the-way spot. That's simple: it's on the equator, so a ship gets the full thousand-mile-an-hour boost of the Earth's spin as it takes off – and there's the whole width of the Pacific for jettisoned fuel tanks to fall into. And if you've ever *heard* a spaceship taking off, you'll understand why the launching sites have to be a few hundred miles from civilization.

Don't be alarmed by anything you've been told about the strain of blast-off. There's really nothing to it if you're in good health – and you won't be allowed inside a spaceship unless you are. You just lie down on the acceleration couch, put in your earplugs, and relax. It takes over a minute for the full thrust to build up, and by that time you're quite accustomed to it. You'll have some difficulty in breathing, perhaps – it's never bothered me – but if you don't attempt to move you'll hardly feel the increase of weight. What you *will* notice is the noise, which is slightly unbelievable. Still, it lasts only five minutes, and by the end of that time you'll be up in orbit and the motors will cut out. Don't worry about your hearing; it will get back to normal in a couple of hours.

You won't see a great deal until you get aboard the space station, because there are no viewing ports on the ferry rockets and passengers aren't encouraged to wander around. It usually takes about thirty minutes to make the necessary steering corrections and to match speed with the station; you'll know when that's happened from the rather alarming 'clang' as the airlocks make contact. Then you can undo your safely belt, and of course you'll want to see what it's like being weightless.

Now, take your time, and do exactly what you're told. Hang on to the guide rope through the airlock and don't try to go flying around like a bird. There'll be plenty of time for that later: there's not enough room in the ferry, and if you attempt any of the usual tricks you'll not only injure yourself but may damage the equipment as well.

Space Station One, which is where the ferries and the liners meet to transfer their cargoes, takes just two hours to make one circuit of the Earth. You'll spend all your time in the observa-tion lounge: everyone does, no matter how many times they've been out into space. I won't attempt to describe that incredible view; I'll merely remind you that in the hundred and twenty minutes it takes the station to complete its orbit you'll see the Earth wax from a thin crescent to a gigantic, multicolored disc, and then shrink again to a black shield eclipsing the stars. As you pass over the night side you'll see the lights of cities down there in the darkness, like patches of phosphorescence. And the stars! You'll realize that you've never really seen them before in your life.

But enough of these purple passages; let's stick to business.

You'll probably remain on Space Station One for about twelve hours, which will give you plenty of opportunity to see how you like weightlessness. It doesn't take long to learn how to move around; the main secret is to avoid all violent motions – otherwise you may crack your head on the ceiling. Except, of course, that there isn't a ceiling since there's no up or down any more. At first you'll find that confusing: you'll have to stop and decide which direction you want to move in, and then adjust your personal reference system to fit. After a few days in space it will be second nature to you.

Don't forget that the station is your last link with Earth. If you want to make any final purchases, or leave something to be sent home – do it then. You won't have another chance for a good many million miles. But beware of buying items that the station shop assures you are 'just the thing on Mars'.

You'll go aboard the liner when you've had your final medical check, and the steward will show you to the little cabin that will be your home for the next few months. Don't be upset because you can touch all the walls without moving from one spot. You'll only have to sleep there, after all, and you've got the rest of the ship to stretch your legs in.

If you're on one of the larger liners, there'll be about a hundred other passengers and a crew of perhaps twenty. You'll get to know them all by the end of the voyage. There's nothing on Earth quite like the atmosphere in a spaceship. You're a little, self-contained community floating in vacuum millions of miles from anywhere, kept alive in a bubble of plastic and metal. If you're a good mixer you'll find the experience very stimulating. But it has its disadvantages. The one great danger of spaceflight is that some prize bore may get on the passenger list – and short of pushing him out of the airlock there's nothing anyone can do about it.

It won't take you long to find your way around the ship and to get used to its gadgets. Handling liquids is the main skill you'll have to acquire: your first attempts at drinking are apt to be messy. Oddly enough, taking a shower is quite simple. You do it in a sort of plastic cocoon, and a circulating air current carries the water out at the bottom.

At first the absence of gravity may make sleeping difficult: you'll miss your accustomed weight. That's why the sheets over the bunks have spring tensioning. They'll keep you from drifting out while you sleep, and their pressure will give you a spurious sensation of weight.

But learning to live under zero gravity is something one can't be taught in advance: you have to find out by experience and practical demonstration. I believe you'll enjoy it, and when the novelty's worn off you'll take it completely for granted. Then the problem will be getting used to gravity again when you reach Mars!

Unlike the take-off of the ferry rocket from Earth, the break-away of the liner from its satellite orbit is so gentle and protracted that it lacks all drama. When the loading and instrument checks have been completed, the ship will uncouple from the Space Station and drift a few miles away. You'll hardly notice it when the atomic drive goes on; there will be the faintest of vibrations and a feeble sensation of weight. The ship's acceleration is so small, in fact, that you'll weigh only a few ounces, which will scarcely interfere with your freedom of movement at all. Its only effect will be to make things drift slowly to one end of the cabin if they're left lying around.

Although the liner's acceleration is so small that it will take hours to break away from Earth and head out into space, after a week of continuous drive the ship will have built up a colossal speed. Then the motors will be cut out and you'll carry on under your own momentum until you reach the orbit of Mars and have to start thinking about slowing down.

Whether your weeks in space are boring or not depends very much on you and your fellow passengers. Quite a number of entertainments get organized on the voyage, and a good deal of money is liable to change hands before the end of the trip. (It's a curious fact, but the crew usually seem to come out on top.) You'll have plenty of time for reading, and the ship will have a good library of microbooks. There will be radio and TV contact with Earth and Mars for the whole voyage, so you'll be able to keep in touch with things – if you want to.

On my first trip, I spent a lot of my time learning my way around the stars and looking at clusters and nebulae through a small telescope I borrowed from the navigation officer. Even if you've never felt the slightest interest in astronomy before, you'll probably be a keen observer before the end of the voyage. Having the stars all around you – not merely overhead – is an experience you'll never forget.

As far as outside events are concerned, you realize, of course, that absolutely nothing can happen during the voyage. Once the drive has cut out, you'll seem to be hanging motionless in space: you'll be no more conscious of your speed than you are of Earth's seventy thousand miles an hour around the Sun right now. The only evidence of your velocity will be the slow movement of the nearer planets against the background of the stars – and you'll have to watch carefully for a good many hours before you can detect even this.

By the way, I hope you aren't one of those foolish people who are still frightened about meteors. They see that enormous chunk of nickel-steel in New York's American Museum of Natural History and imagine that's the sort of thing you'll run smack into as soon as you leave the atmosphere – forgetting that there's rather a lot of room in space and that even the biggest ship is a mighty small target. You'd have to sit out there and wait a good many centuries before a meteor big enough to puncture the hull came along. It hasn't happened to a spaceship yet.

One of the big moments of the trip will come when you realize that Mars has begun to show a visible disc. The first feature you'll be able to see with the naked eye will be one of the polar caps, glittering like a tiny star on the edge of the planet. A few days later the dark areas – the so-called seas – will begin to appear, and presently you'll glimpse the prominent triangle of Syrtis Major. In the week before landing, as the planet swims nearer and nearer, you'll get to know its geography pretty thoroughly.

The braking period doesn't last very long, as the ship has lost a good deal of its speed in the climb outward from the Sun. When it's over you'll be dropping down onto Phobos, the inner moon of Mars, which acts as a natural space station about four thousand miles above the surface of the planet. Though Phobos is only a jagged lump of rock not much bigger than some terrestrial mountains, it's reassuring to be in contact with something solid again after so many weeks in space.

When the ship has settled down into the landing cradle, the airlock will be coupled up and you'll go through a connecting tube into the port. Since Phobos is much too small to have an appreciable gravity, you'll still be effectively weightless. While the ship's being unloaded the immigration officials will check your papers. I don't know the point of this; I've never heard of anyone being sent all the way back to Earth after having got this far!

There are two things you mustn't miss at Port Phobos. The restaurant there is quite good, even though the food is largely synthetic; it's very small, and only goes into action when a liner docks, but it does its best to give you a fine welcome to Mars. And after a couple of months you'll have got rather tired of the shipboard menu.

The other item is the centrifuge; I believe that's compulsory now. You go inside and it will spin you up to half a gravity, or rather more than the weight Mars will give you when you land. It's simply a little cabin on a rotating arm, and there's room to walk around inside so that you can practise using your legs again. You probably won't like the feeling; life in a spaceship can make you lazy.

The ferry rockets that will take you down to Mars will be waiting when the ship docks. If you're unlucky you'll hang around at the port for some hours, because they can't carry more than twenty passengers and there are only two ferries in service. The actual descent to the planet takes about three hours, and it's the only time on the whole trip when you'll get any impression of speed. Those ferries enter the atmosphere at over five thousand miles an hour and go halfway around Mars before they lose enough speed through air resistance to land like ordinary aircraft.

You'll land, of course, at Port Lowell: besides being the largest settlement on Mars it's still the only place that has the facilities for handling spaceships. From the air the plastic pressure domes look like a cluster of bubbles – a very pretty sight when the Sun catches them. Don't be alarmed if one of them is deflated. That doesn't mean that there's been an accident. The domes are let down at fairly frequent intervals so that the envelopes can be checked for leaks. If you're lucky you may see one being pumped up – it's quite impressive.

After two months in a spaceship, even Port Lowell will seem a mighty metropolis. (Actually, I believe its population is now well over twenty thousand.) You'll find the people energetic, inquisitive, forthright – and very friendly, unless they think you're trying to be superior.

It's a good working rule never to criticize anything you see on Mars. As I said before, they're very proud of their achievements and after all you *are* a guest, even if a paying one.

Port Lowell has practically everything you'll find in a city on Earth, though of course on a smaller scale. You'll come across many reminders of 'home'. For example, the main street in the city is Fifth Avenue – but surprisingly enough you'll find Piccadilly Circus where it crosses Broadway.

The port, like all the major settlements, lies in the dark belt of vegetation that roughly follows the equator and occupies about half the southern hemisphere. The northern hemisphere is almost all desert – the red oxides that give the planet its ruddy colour. Some of these desert regions are very beautiful; they're far older than anything on the surface of our Earth, because there's been little weathering on Mars to wear down the rocks – at least since the seas dried up, more than 500 million years ago.

You shouldn't attempt to leave the city until you've become quite accustomed to living in an oxygen-rich, low-pressure atmosphere. You'll have grown fairly well acclimatized on the trip, because the air in the spaceship will have been slowly adjusted to conditions on Mars. Outside the domes, the pressure of the natural Martian atmosphere is about equal to that on the top of Mount Everest* – and it contains practically no oxygen. So when you go out you'll have to wear a helmet, or travel in one of those pressurized jeeps they call 'sand fleas'.

Wearing a helmet, by the way, is nothing like the nuisance you'd expect it to be. The equipment is very light and compact and, as long as you don't do anything silly, is quite foolproof. As it's very unlikely that you'll ever go out without an experienced guide, you'll have no need to worry. Thanks to the low gravity, enough oxygen for twelve hours' normal working can be carried quite easily – and you'll never be away from shelter as long as that.

Don't attempt to imitate any of the locals you may see walking around without oxygen gear. They're second-generation colonists and are used to the low pressure. They can't breathe the Martian atmosphere any more than you can, but like the old-time native pearl divers they can make one lungful last for several minutes when necessary. Even so, it's a silly sort of trick and they're not supposed to do it.

As you know, the other great obstacle to life on Mars is the low temperature. The highest thermometer reading ever recorded is somewhere in the eighties, but that's quite exceptional. In the long winters, and during the night in summer *or* winter, it never rises above freezing. And I believe the record low is minus one hundred and ninety!

Well, you won't be outdoors at night, and for the sort of excursions you'll be doing, all that's needed is a simple thermosuit. It's very light, and traps the body heat so effectively that no other source of warmth is needed.

No doubt you'll want to see as much of Mars as you can during your stay. There are only two methods of transport outside the cities – sand fleas for short ranges and aircraft for longer distances. Don't misunderstand me when I say 'short ranges' – a sand flea with a full charge of power cells is good for a couple of thousand miles, and it can do eighty miles an hour over good ground. Mars could never have been explored without them. You can *survey* a planet from space, but in the end someone with a pick and shovel has to do the dirty work filling in the map.

One thing that few visitors realize is just how *big* Mars is. Although it seems small beside the Earth, its land area is almost as great because so much of our planet is covered with oceans. So it's hardly surprising that there are vast regions that have never been properly explored, particularly around the poles. Those stubborn people who still believe that there was once an indigenous Martian civilization pin their hopes on these great blanks. Every so often you hear rumours of some wonderful archaeological discovery in the wastelands, but nothing ever comes of it.

Personally, I don't believe there ever *were* any Martians – but the planet is interesting enough for its own sake. You'll be fascinated by the plant life and the queer animals that manage to live without oxygen, migrating each year from hemisphere to hemisphere, across the ancient sea beds, to avoid the ferocious winter.

The fight for survival on Mars has been fierce, and evolution has produced some pretty odd results. Don't go investigating any Martian lifeforms unless you have a guide, or you may get some unpleasant surprises. Some plants are so hungry for heat that they may try to wrap themselves around you.

Well, that's all I've got to say, except to wish you a pleasant trip. Oh, there *is* one other thing. My boy collects stamps, and I rather let him down when I was on Mars. If you could drop me a few letters while you're there – there's no need to put anything in them if you're too busy – I'd be much obliged. He's trying to collect a set of space-mail covers postmarked from all the Martian Cities, and if you could help – thanks a lot!

*This estimate, we now know, is more than ten times too high.

Further Reading

Chapter 1: Prelude to Mars

Lowell's own books have long been out of print and are not readily available: I am extremely grateful to the National Geographic Society's senior editor (and pioneer underwater explorer) Luis Marden for my copy of *Mars as the Abode of Life* (Macmillan, 1910). However, all that one needs to know about the Lowellian delusion will be found in:

1. *Lowell and Mars*: William Graves Hoyt (University of Arizona Press, 1976).
2. *Planets and Perception*: William Sheenan (University of Arizona Press, 1988).

Chapter 3: Going There

The literature, both popular and technical, on methods of reaching Mars is now enormous. In addition to the International Space University study described from page 34 onwards, the following are of particular interest:

1. 'EMPIRE: Early Manned Planetary–Interplanetary Round-trip Expeditions': Frederick I. Ordway III, Mitchell R. Sharpe and Ronald C. Wakeford (*Journal of the British Interplanetary Society*, vol 46 no 5, May 1993).

Even while the *Apollo* program was getting underway, Dr Wernher von Braun assigned members of his team to plan expeditions to Mars and Venus, and study contracts were issued to Ford's Aeronutronic Division, General Dynamics and Lockheed. It was concluded that Saturn-V launch vehicles and the NERVA nuclear rocket then under development would allow manned missions to the two planets in the early 1970s.

2. *Space Transfer Concepts and Analysis for Exploration Missions*: Boeing Defense and Space Group (Huntsville, Alabama, Contract NAS8-37857, December 1991). Summarized in *New Mars Vehicle Concepts* by Brent Sherwood (AIAA Paper 93–1069).

3. 'Mars Direct: Humans to the Red Planet by 1999': Robert M. Zubrin and David A. Baker (*Acta Astronautica*, vol 26 no 12, pp 899–912, December 1992).

The Boeing study (a detailed 218-page report) analyses all currently known propulsion systems, including nuclear, for missions in the AD2014–16 period. 'Mars Direct', a study by two engineers at Martin Marietta, is much more speculative (not to say optimistic, as indicated by its title!). Only chemical propulsion is used in the first phase, in which an automated return vehicle is landed on Mars and manufactures propellants (methane/oxygen) from local resources.

4. *America at the Threshold*: Synthesis Group (US Government Printing Office, Washington DC, 1991).
5. *Exploring the Moon and Mars: Choices for the Nation*: US Congress, Office of Technology Assessment (US Government Printing Office, Washington DC, 1991).

These two studies were published in response to President Bush's 1989 'Space Exploration Initiative' (SEI), in which he spoke about returning to the Moon 'to stay' and landing on Mars by the fiftieth anniversary of *Apollo* 11 (i.e., 2019). The Synthesis Group, headed by astronaut Thomas Stafford, outlined plans for putting humans on the Moon by AD2003–5 and on Mars by AD2014–16.

6. 'International Manned Missions to Mars and the Resources of Phobos and Deimos': Brian O'Leary (*Acta Astronautica*, vol 26 no 1, pp 37–54, 1992).

This stimulating paper was presented at the Thirty-Ninth Congress of the International Astronautical Federation, Bangalore, India, in 1988. Dr O'Leary proposed a mission to the Martian satellites in 1998–9 by adapting one of the US Shuttle's external tanks as a mission module transfer vehicle. He assumes from their density and reflectivity that Phobos and Deimos are similar to carbonaceous meteorites, which contain ten to twenty per cent water. If this is the case, and it can be extracted by solar or nuclear energy, thousands of tons of water could be delivered to the surface of Mars and the Moon by 2005. Martian and lunar bases could then be established, and 'a space industrial infrastructure could grow rapidly for other space development scenarios'.

This timescale seems highly optimistic – especially since the failure of the *Phobos* (USSR) and *Mars Observer* (United States) missions, whose inputs would have been essential to the scenario. But there can be little doubt that Mars' two tiny satellites will play a role in the planet's exploration quite out of proportion to their size.

Dr O'Leary has also published a book on this theme: *Mars 1999* (Stackpole Books, Harrisburg, Pa., 1987).

7. 'Fast Track to Mars': Hans Mark and Harlan J. Smith (*Aerospace America*, August 1992).

Dr Mark (Past Deputy Administrator, NASA) and his colleagues at the University of Texas, Austin, argue that it would be possible to return to the Moon by 1995 using the existing Shuttle and Titan-IV launch vehicles: the main purpose of the mission would be to look for ice near the lunar poles: 'A wet Moon would mean the trip to Mars would start from lunar rather than Earth orbit . . . launch to Mars would occur in early 2003 and the first landing in October 2003.' Unmanned, solar-powered ion rockets would fly preliminary cargo missions.

8. *The Case for Mars*: a series of important volumes published by the American Astronautical Society (vol I, 1984; vol II, 1985; vol III, 1987).

Most of the papers are technical, but the 'Mars II Conference' (University of Colorado, 10–14 July 1984) contains a challenging essay, 'A Timeline for Martian Pioneers', by Thomas O. Paine (1921–92), NASA Administrator during the key years of the *Apollo* program, 1968–70. A later version, 'To Settle the Red Planet: A Decade-by-Decade Look at Martian History, 1990 to 2090', was published in the Planetary Society's special tribute to Dr Paine (*The Planetary Report*, vol XII no 5, September/October 1992). Some highlights from Tom Paine's 'History' are:

○ 2000–2010: Return to the Moon. Shuttle fleet retired after 'another tragic accident'. Martian habitats tested on the Moon.

○ 2010–2020: First humans land on Mars.

○ 2020–2030: Nuclear power plants separate oxygen and hydrogen from Martian permafrost to fuel surface transport and surface-to-orbit shuttles. Birth of first Martian baby.

○ 2030–2040: Build-up of Mars bases; population several hundred.

○ 2040–2050: Lunar-demonstrated robotic agriculture reducing costly dependence on Earth. Population 1000.

○ 2050–2060: Build-up of mass-less interplanetary trade depending on artificial intelligence and software communication to robotic factories ('virtual teleportation'). Population 5000.

○ 2060–2070: Resources of asteroids and outer planets being explored: Mars heading for self-sufficiency. Other galactic civilizations detected by Mars–Earth interferometers. Population 10,000 humans + 100,000 equivalent robots.

○ 2070–2080: Tourism and immigration builds up population to 50,000. Matter–antimatter drive developed for space propulsion.

○ 2080–2090: The vigorous young Mars settlements contain 100,000 people and close to 1 million equivalent robots. Martian immigration policy is promoting a rich gene pool from every continent on Earth, while biological laboratories, zoos, gene libraries, museums, art galleries, and book and image libraries house extensive collections of terrestrial life. Although a lively trade is under way, the continuation of life on Mars no longer depends upon imports from Earth; the same is true of the Moon. Martians, Lunarians and Earthlings are now evolving independently on three resource-rich worlds.

Genetically engineered bacteria are under test to initiate the terraforming of Venus and Mars. Young Martians are pressing for additional settlements beyond the asteroid belt, and in response promising sites on Triton, Titan and other moons of Uranus, Saturn and Jupiter are being surveyed. Joint Mars–Earth–Moon research on matter–antimatter and photon propulsion to drive spacecraft at speeds approaching ten per cent of the speed of light shows promise of opening the challenging 'stellar frontier'. And, finally, long-range plans call for launching robotic probes to temperate planets circling nearby stars before the end of the century.

And if anyone considers that this scenario is 'mere' science fiction, let me emphasize that these were the considered thoughts, at the end of his life, of the man who directed the greatest engineering feat in history: the first landing by human beings on another celestial body.

9. *Space Resources*: edited by Mary Fae McKay, David S. McKay and Michael B. Duke (NASA SP–509: US Government Printing Office, 1992).

This massive, lavishly illustrated four-volume set covers every aspect of space exploration and colonization, including the mining of the Moon and the asteroids, extraterrestrial bases and eventually 'sightseeing'. Who would have imagined, even a few decades ago, that a US Government publication (vol 1: *Scenarios*) would conclude: 'Other optimistic visions of the future of space activities might include extensive tourism . . . The idea that much of the Solar System might eventually be available for anyone to visit is clearly a visionary one, but one that is not beyond the reach of projected advances in technology.'

The literature about *living* on Mars must now be as extensive as that concerned with getting there. Some convenient references are:

10. 'Engineering and Technology for a Mars Base': *Journal of the British Interplanetary Society* (vol 45 no 5, May 1992).

Contains five papers on 'Mars Solar Energy Systems', 'Exploration Strategies and the Astronaut's Toolset', 'Long Range Mobility', 'An Internal Combustion (Otto-Cycle) Engine on Mars' and 'Space Suits and Life Support Systems'.

11. *Pioneering the Space Frontier*: The Report of the National Commission on Space (Bantam Books, New York, 1986).

12. *Planetary Exploration through the Year 2000*: NASA Advisory Council (US Government Printing Office, Washington DC, 1986).

13. 'Pioneering Mars': Robert Zubrin and Chris McKay (*Ad Astra*, vol 4 no 6, September/October 1992).

This whole issue of the magazine of the National Space Society (922, Pennsylvania Avenue SE, Washington DC) is devoted to Mars, and contains some excellent illustrations.

Chapter 5: The Snows of Olympus
Long after writing this chapter I came across Brian Aldiss' short story 'The Difficulties in Photographing Nix Olympica' (in the collection *Best SF Stories of Brian W. Aldiss* [1988]). I could not help telling Brian that from ground-level it was not merely difficult – it was impossible.

Chapter 8: The Longest Spring
1. 'What About the Environmental Statement? The Law and Ethics of Terraforming': Glenn H. Reynolds (*Ad Astra*, vol 4 no 6, September/October 1992).

Article IX of the UN's Outer Space Treaty obliges its signatories to avoid activities that will result in the 'harmful contamination' of the Moon and other celestial bodies. Defining this may be difficult – especially if we discover extraterrestrial life.

2. 'Making Mars Habitable': Christopher P. McKay, Owen B. Toon and James F. Kasting (*Nature*, vol 352 no 6335, 8 August 1991).

This important paper (eight pages with eighty-three references) was probably the first introduction that many scientists outside the space community had to the idea of terraforming, and the fact that it appeared in *Nature* compelled them to take it seriously.

3. 'Terraforming': *Journal of the British Interplanetary Society* (vol 45 no 8, August 1992).

This contains two papers which come to widely differing conclusions. 'A Synergetic Approach to Terraforming Mars' by Martyn J. Fogg proposes the use of 'greenhouse gases' (fluorocarbons), among other technologies, to warm the planet and release frozen water and carbon dioxide. Mars might then be able to support hardy microbes and plant life in about 200 years – but it would require 21,000 years before conditions would be tolerable to human beings . . . By contrast, 'Terraforming Mars Quickly' by Paul Birch suggests that by using large orbital mirrors ('solettas') it might be possible to warm the planet so rapidly that it became habitable in as little as fifty years! Both authors would probably agree that the trifling discrepancy in their calculations cannot be resolved until we know vastly more about Mars and its resources than we do today.

4. *The Greening of Mars* by Michael Allaby & James Lovelock (Andre Deutsch, London 1984).

Co-authored by the originator of the Gaia Hypothesis, and

written from the point of view of a second-generation Martian colonist looking back (often critically) at Earth–Mars politics. Although the suggested scenario – first landing May 1997, sponsored by a private consortium which bought up the ex-Cold War rockets and adapted them to deliver the equally unwanted 'greenhouse gases' (freon, etc.) on Mars! – now seems rather naïve, this short novel is full of wisdom and is well worth reading.

5. I cannot resist quoting this letter, which appeared in the *New York Times* for 22 October 1991:

Be Certain Mars Has No Dinosaurs

The project to make Mars habitable by terraforming should not be ridiculed, as some scientists are doing ('Can Mars Be Made Hospitable to Humans?', *Science Times*, October 1). Its proponents would warm up the red planet by creating a greenhouse effect.

This is in fact the way Earth was made habitable. An econometric model prepared on Venus in approximately 200,000,000BC has recently been discovered in a cave in Colorado and is now being analysed in our university's computers.

Faced with the problem of their own planet becoming uninhabitable through irreversible global warming, Venusian economists calculated the costs and benefits of heating up a barren Earth. The exact path of economic and social development was charted, including the evolution of democracy, socialism, and the size of government deficits. When all this had been done, a massive space lift brought the inhabitants of Venus to Earth.

Unfortunately, they were all eaten by dinosaurs, and human evolution had to start again.

The moral: No econometric model is perfect.

JOHN P. POWELSON
Professor of Econometrics,
University of Colorado, Boulder, Colorado.
4 October 1991

Need I say that some readers, brain-damaged by the mental junk food on their local news-stands, wrote to Professor Powelson asking for the location of the Colorado cave?

Acknowledgements

First of all, my thanks to John Hinkley, whose Vistapro program made this book possible, and who flew out to Sri Lanka to install it and to supercharge my Amiga.

Also to Dr R. M. Batson, Planetary Cartography Section of the US Geological Survey, Flagstaff, for sending me masses of cartographic material on Mars.

And to Robert L. Millis, Director of the Lowell Observatory, and to Richard Bolin, Chairman of the Observatory Board, for general assistance and providing many of the illustrations.

To Nick Veitch and his colleagues at Future Publishing for downloading images from my tapes.

To my long-time friend and colleague Fred Durant, Space Art International, for locating artwork and obtaining permissions at a moment's notice.

And especially to Paul Barnett (a.k.a. John Grant), who, although he eviscerated much of my deathless prose and removed my favourite jokes, did a remarkable job of editing the manuscript and, above all, sorting out and recaptioning the illustrations.

Finally, my gratitude for inspiration provided by several generations of space artists – going back to the great Chesley Bonestell, who started it all. I hope this book continues the tradition . . .

Index

Page numbers in **bold** refer to relevant captions